THE
MALE
MEMBER

THE
MALE
MEMBER

*Being a Compendium
of Facts, Figures,
Foibles, and Anecdotes
about the Loving Organ*

KIT SCHWARTZ

ST. MARTIN'S PRESS

NEW YORK

Design by M. Paul

Library of Congress Cataloging in Publication Data

Schwartz, Kit.
The male member.

1. Penis—Miscellanea.   2. Penis—Anecdotes, facetiae,
satire, etc.   I. Title.
QP257.S39   1985   591.4'6   85-1850
ISBN 0-312-50933-2

First Edition

10 9 8 7 6 5 4 3 2 1

TO
SAM SCHWARTZ
(clink)

CONTENTS

Acknowledgments   ix
Preface   xi

1 Penis Has Personality Plus   1
Descriptions and definitions of the penis and the
male genital area that have come down through
the ages from many cultures.

2 You've Got that Thing   13
Describing and locating the penises of various animals and insects. A report on a unique penis, the
autosexual's. A historical survey of the phallic
symbol.

3 Manual Pollution and the "Big M" Plague   20
Ancient taboos against male masturbation. Religion versus masturbation. The Big M plague:
Science discovers masturbation and comes to
grips with it. The statistical solution for masturbation.

4 Erogeny—A Beginning to Make Both Ends Meet   32
What, since the beginning of life, turns a penis up?

5 Nipping in the Bud   47
You're damned if you do and damned if you
don't—dumping an orgasm, is it waste?

6 "You Used to Come at 4 O'clock, and Now You Come at
Noon!" 54
Aphrodisiacs and anaphrodisiacs from many ages
and cultures.

7 Thrust Not or Forever Hold Your Piece 74
The history of sexual abstinence and celibacy.

8 Castration Complexity 92
The categories and degrees of male castration. Eunuchs and how they coped—from ancient times to
the present. The history and anatomy of transsexuality. What about those animals made eunuchs
by humans?

9 Man the Pump, the Penis Is Inflamed 109
The history of gonorrhea and syphilis. The origin
of the condom remains a mystery—why? Has genital herpes KO'ed a revolution? Some straight talk
about AIDS.

10 The Penile Colony 131
The choky etymological history of homosexuality.

11 The Adventure of the Odd Ball and Other Bones of
Contention 151
Mysterious male genitals that stick out to this
day.

12 The Penis Explodes into the Twenty-first Century 169
Future possibilities for the male genitals—some in
the works, some a pipe dream.

Bibliography 182
Index 189

ACKNOWLEdGMENTS

Thank you, Robert Hughes, for editing the penis; Elizabeth Crown for the medical checkups on the penis; Eugene Wildman for cheering the penis on; and Carol Baldwin for her in-depth research on the penis.

Also, in grateful memory, to George Buehr for arousing my curiosity about the penis as he cranked out penile tales while we toured the back roads of Europe.

I am also indebted to the Kinsey Institute for Sex Research, Bloomington, Indiana; the Playboy library, Chicago, Illinois; the American Medical Association library, Chicago; the New York Public Library; the Newberry Library, Chicago; the private medical library of Dr. Miodrag Mihailovic; and Dr. Joseph H. Kiefer's collection of the history of urology in the Department of the Library of Health Sciences, the University of Illinois at Chicago.

And, finally, a big hand to John Santucci, who supported the penis to its climactic conclusion.

pREfACE

The Male Member is a quick study, speed-reading, sex history course uncovering the penis of the male animal. This book is filled with factual historical descriptions of the varieties in male sexual practices, and the similarities and differences between human and animal sexual behavior. It is a Who, What, When, Where, and sometimes Why book of male sexuality from the perspective of the penis, from the prehistoric to the now.

What are some of the things a reader could learn in the course of reading this book?

Looking back at various sexual practices of many nations and cultures through history, the reader will find that standards and methods go up and down and switch around and around; that a kangaroo's penis is backward (in structure, not ability); that Chinese eunuchs pickled their penises and then presented them to would-be employers as a résumé; that in some cultures women could have their eyes torn out for damaging a male's testicles during a domestic quarrel (an eye for a ball); that in ancient Greece, kidnapping young males was a form of homosexual courtship; and that certain men—not necessarily double-jointed—are able to have anal sex with themselves.

Is this book definitive?

By no means! A sequel is already in the works, for sex

has two superstars—the penis and the vagina. Or so it was when this book went to press.

As for this attempt to peg the penis: we hope that when all has been said and read, the penis will be put in its proper place.

Kit Schwartz

1

PENIS HAS PERSONALITY PLUS

The penis of man is located below the navel, at the top of the thighs, and within arm's reach. Since it visibly alters in appearance and activity with a change in mood, many consider the penis to have a personality and spirit of its own. And so diverse are these alterations, one might well compare them with the switch from the placid (flaccid) Dr. Jekyll to the aggressive (rampant) Mr. Hyde.

For the most part, the penis acts the role of the more conventional Dr. Jekyll—a retiring figure with an indifferent attitude. His posture is noticeably slack, and his skin has a spongy texture that hangs loose. His size is nothing great; he averages between

3¼ and 4¼ inches in length and about 3⅜ inches in circumference.

But it's a whole new ball game when Dr. Jekyll gets his hit—a rush of blood from an erotic arousal. He becomes the assertive Mr. Hyde with a decidedly upward, mobile, and outgoing attitude. His posture firms to West Point perfect. His skin tightens and glistens. His head gets a ruddy glow. His mouth wears a little smile. He is very popular and he rarely overstays his welcome.

Erotic texts from ancient India claim there is a definite relationship between the size of the penis in erection and the destiny and general configuration of its owner. The *Ananga Ranga* in the sixteenth century declared that the owners of thin penises would be lucky. Fated to be poor were those with very long ones (that's why money isn't everything). Males with thick penises were doomed always to be distressed (wanna bet?), while those with short ones could become rulers of the land (now guess what size the author of the *Ananga Ranga* had).

Further back in time, somewhere around the fourth century, the erotic manual the *Kama Sutra* declared that erect penises come in three different sizes and flavors and that they can be identified by the general physique and disposition of their owners. For instance, penis number 1 does not exceed five inches during erection and has semen with a sweetish flavor. The owner is short of stature but well built and has a quiet disposition. This penis is considered one of small dimension and has been nicknamed the Hare.

Penis number 2 does not exceed seven inches. Since the flavor of this penis is not mentioned in the translation, we can only assume it to be innocuous. The owner of number 2 is described as usually robust, with a high forehead, large eyes, a restless temperament, and always eager to do it. This penis is considered of middle dimension and is nicknamed the Bull (quite a jump from the Hare).

Penis number 3 is a lengthy ten inches. And the owner of this mighty implement is (from a translation made by Nik Douglas in *Sexual Secrets*): "Usually tall, large-framed, muscular and has a deep voice. His nature is gluttonous, covetous, passionate, reckless and lazy. He walks slowly and cares little for love making, unless suddenly overcome by desire. His semen is copious and usually rather salty. He is known as being of *large dimension*." His nickname is the Horse.

At this moment the longest penis ever recorded is a strained thirteen inches.

A recent businesslike sex manual, *Human Sex Anatomy*, pragmatically reports that the size of the penis has less relationship to general body size than that of other organs of the body. But the same does not necessarily hold true when it comes to the color of the skin. Dr. Lonny Myers, who has performed countless vasectomies, claims that of one hundred black-, white-, and yellow-skinned penises, among the black-skinned there would be a bigger percentage of large penises than in the white-skinned, and that the white-skinned would have a bigger percentage of large members than the yellow-skinned.

The ancient Chinese preferred to describe the nature of the penis by its behavior. Take this quote from *The Prayer Cushion of the Flesh:*

> At night it was very different; then his naughty, his sinful, his mutinous henchman did everything it could to attract attention. Under the coarse wool blanket it would stretch and sprawl, rise up in defiance, or saunter haughtily about. Lord in Heaven, how impetuously his external disturber of the peace had risen up, how conspicuous his rebellious henchman was making himself! All stiff and proud, it could be seen holding up a blanket with its head; peering eastward and leering westward, obviously searching for one of its customary hiding places.

The classical Arabian book on physical love, *The Perfumed Garden*, also prefers to describe the character of the penis from its actions. This book, translated by Sir Richard Burton, gives a listing of thirty word portraits. Here are a few that have risen for the occasion:

> The Housebreaker—On coming to the door of the vulva, this one is asked, "What do you want?" "I want to come in!" the Housebreaker replies. "Impossible! I cannot take you in on account of your size."
>
> Then the member insists that the other one should only receive its head, promising not to come in entirely; it then approaches, rubs its head twice or thrice between the vulva's lips, till they get humid and thus lubricated, then introduces first its head, and after, with one push, plunges in up to the testicles.
>
> The Impudent—has received this name because from the moment that it gets stiff and long it does not care for anybody, lifts impudently the clothing of its master by raising its head fiercely, and makes him ashamed while it itself feels no shame. It acts in the same unabashed way with women, turning up their clothes and laying bare their thighs. Its master may blush at this conduct, but as to itself, its stiffness and determination to plunge into the vulva only increase.
>
> The Weeper—So called on account of the many tears it sheds; as soon as it gets an erection, it weeps; when it sees a pretty face, it weeps; handling a woman, it weeps. It goes even so far as to weep tears sacred to memory.
>
> The Stumbler—It is called so because if it wants to penetrate the vulva, as it does not see the door, it beats about above and below, and thus continues to stumble as over stones in the road, until the lips of the vulva get humid, when it manages to get inside. The vulva then says, "What has happened to you that made you stumble about so?" The member answers, "O my love, it was a stone lying in the road."
>
> The Sleeper—from its deceitful appearance. When it gets into erection, it lengthens out and stiffens itself

to such an extent that one might think it would never get soft again. But when it has left the vulva, after having satisfied its passion, it goes to sleep.

There are members that fall asleep while inside the vulva, but the majority of them come out still firm; but at that moment they get drowsy, and little by little fall asleep.

Still another Chinese description of the penis comes from the *Linga Purana*, written during the late Ming Dynasty. This penis has it all, for it is:

Beautiful as molten gold, firm as the Himalaya Mountain, tender as a folded leaf, life-giving like the solar orb; behold the charm of his sparkling jewels!

In Western cultures since the Age of Enlightenment, descriptions of the penis have become mostly anatomical. Here is a 1982 version given by urologist Sherman J. Silber in his book *The Male:*

The penis is basically composed of three parallel cylinders, all enclosed in an outer sheath of very stretchable, elastic skin. The two major cylinders . . . extend all of the way down to the bone we sit on. An erect penis is thus supported by a firm foundation. Without this . . . the penis would wobble around and buckle during the in and out motions of intercourse. A third cylinder surrounds the urethra, [where] . . . the urine and the semen squirt out.

There are exceptions, of course, to the Western world's predilection for scientific descriptions of the male sexual organ. One that dates back to the turn of the century is from a European named Captain Charles Devereaux. His book, *Venus in India*, was considered pornographic during Victorian time. Here is the Captain's bald portrait of the penis:

"Give me your hand!" He took it and put it on what felt like a great big thick stick, thicker than a broom handle, and hot and awfully hard, except for the outside, which felt like velvet, and which was loose and moveable. It was so big that I could hardly get my fingers round it. The very feel of it, however, made my brain whirl around.

The most succinct contemporary definition of the penis comes from the twenty-first printing of *The Compact Edition of the Oxford English Dictionary* (June 1981): "The intromittent or copulatory organ of any male animal (in Mammalia also transversed by the urethra)."

What the English-speaking world loses in poetry it makes up for in the limitless pet names that have come down through the centuries. Most of these nicknames are complimentary, others a definite put-down. Here is an extensive, though far from exhaustive, list divided into twenty-two categories to emphasize the multifaceted personality of the human penis and other male genitalia.

SACRED OBJECT	DIGNITARY
Saint Peter	Solicitor general
Yang pagoda	Big man on campus
Rector of the females	Scepter
Monk	Seat of strength
Holy sacrament	My captain's body
Priapus	Privy member
Father confessor	General
Holy poker	Diplomat
Holy Kee-rist!	Kingpin
One of the nine gates of the	Ambassador
Holy City	Hero
	Big honcho

DIGNITARY (*cont'd.*)

Captain Standish
Aaron's rod
Julius Caesar
Peacemaker
Quartermaster

GOVERNMENT ISSUE

Privates
Washington Monument
Short arm
Warrior
Lance
Ramrod
Potent regiment
Pistol
Semiautomatic
Weapon
Cutlass
Bayonet
Cannon balls and cannon
Bullet
Cracksman
Battering piece
Sword
Trigger

RENEGADE

Firebrand
Rebellious henchman
Ruffian
Assailant

RENEGADE (*cont'd.*)

External disturber of the
  peace
Mutinous member
Jezebel
Fucker
Unruly member

TREASURE

Pillar of ivory
Family jewels
Bootleg
Gem
The precious
Jade scepter
Grand masterpiece
Magic wand
Pride and joy
Golddigger
Lamp of life

FRIEND

Old blind Bob
Faithful servant
John Thomas
Old Horny
Dickety, Dickety Dick
My boy
Mr. Nicefoot
Auld Hornie
My doodle
Richard

FRIEND (cont'd.)

Roger and out
My Jack
Johnson
Old Slimy

AUTO PARTS

Headlight
Pistol rod
Tailpipe
The engine
Hotrod
Dip-stick

ENTERTAINMENT

Merrymaker
Plaything
Joy knob
Lip-splitter
The jet set
Bubblehead
Front and center
Perker-upper
Hokey-poker
Stud poker
Tickler
Do-funny
Ladies' Delight
Lullaby
Wazoo

ROMANTIC

Thumb of love
My affair
Dart of Venus
Spear of love
Cupid's torch

NATURE BOY

Bald-headed root
Thorn in the flesh
Wringling pole
Hermit in a cave
My stalk
Mountain
Bush beater
Cherry picker
Stem
Hayburner
Ballock-stones
Long arrow
Crack hunter
Vigorous peak
Nature's masterpiece
Sting
Poon-tagger
Pioneer
Tent peg
Whip
Husband of Nature
Nature's scythe
Plum tree shaker
A strong stump between my
    thighs

ANIMALS

Hot fish
Goose's neck
Codpiece
Serpent
Live rabbit
Proud courser
Eel
Steed
Cock
Pecker
Goldfish
Bull
Tail
Flying dick
Pants rabbit
Frog
Tiger
Crimson bird
Cockerel
Unicorn
Beak
Snake in the grass
Mouse
Cuckoo
Sponge
Lizard
Dragon
Worm

HARDWARE

Prick
Tool

HARDWARE (*cont'd.*)

Yard measure
Point
Instrument
Grinding tool
Pump
Hoe handle
Reamer
Plug
Plowshare
Knob
Extension cord
The blade
Boner
Pego
Arse wedge
Grunt iron
Implement
Lead joint
Screwdriver
Prong
Jerking iron
Pikestaff
Pendulum
Nine-inch knocker
Wire
Flying blowtorch

FOODS

Hambone
Gravy giver
Honey pot
Yum-yum
Drumstick

FOODS (cont'd.)
Radish
Lollipop
Marrow-bone and cleaver
Sausage
Carrot
Bag boy
Fruit-ful
Big banana
Egghead
Meat
Hot pudding
Juice dealer
Meat and pickles
Creamstick
Various elongated vegetables
    (and longer is better)

SINNER

The carnal part
Fornicator
Whore pipe

MUSICAL INSTRUMENT

Flute
Pipe organ
Horn
Bell rope
Fiddle bow
Ding-dong

PLAYING DOCTOR

Blue skin
Pulse
Phallus
Seminal vesicles
Pudendum
Erogenous zone
Prostate
Groin
Scrotum
Penile
Foreskin
Proboscis
Genitalia
Sex organ
Vasa deferentia
Rump splitter
Reproductive system after
    puberty
Arse opener
Gonads
Sexual response zone
Prepuce
Orifice
Glans
Epididymides
Lung disturber
Kidney scraper

RECREATIONAL AREAS

Balloon room
Balls and the jack

RECREATIONAL AREAS (cont'd.)

A bag of tricks
The spunk
Jerktown
Bum and balls
A floater
Jack in the box

HOUSEHOLD ITEMS

Chink stopper
Broom handle
Butter knife
Candle
Percolator
Pencil with a tassel
Button hole worker
Teapot
Spindle
Hose
Knocker
Clothes prop
Water spout
Rolling pin

PRACTICALITIES

Dildo
Know-it-all
Lead pipe clincher
Nice little piece of
    possibility
Do-gooder
Got the point

PRACTICALITIES (cont'd.)

Best leg of three
1-2-3 and a splash
Hard-up
My sack
Organ of generation
Scepter of his means
Well-hung
Adept
Outsmart
Kit and caboodle
Life preserver
Skyscraper
End piece
Red cap
Whanger
Frigamajig
Dingus
Gap stopper
Girlometer
Sexing piece
Milkman
Pilgrim's stuff
Schlonge
Quim wedge
Baby maker
Cranny hunter
Irish roots
Pile driver

A WEIRDO!

Dagger
Bludgeon club
Weapon

11

A WIERDO! (*cont'd.*)

Spear of love
Battering ram
Archfiend
The club
A crook

BODY PIECES

Muscle of love
The nose
Joint
Little finger
Pisser
Roly-poly
Forefinger
Body's captain
Pimple

A DUMMY

Dingbat
Dribbling dart of love
Dum-dum
Flip-flop
Peewee
The nag
Fool sticker
Gentle tittler
Giggle stick
Goober
Hang up Johnny
Wigga-waggs
Stumper
Slug
Schmuck
Nuthouse
Greenhorn

2

YOU'VE GOT THAT THING

The penis is land-, sea- and air-borne. Geographically the penis can be located with small effort in most areas of the world, yet on the body, it's not always obvious to the eye.

For instance the kangaroo's penis is tucked behind his testicles, while the penis of a dragonfly is hidden in his stomach. The mosquito's penis is another one difficult to light upon, for during courtship while in flight, his lower abdomen rotates 180 degrees, which, anatomically, points his organ down side up. Sneakier still is the sex organ of the bat, as it moves by itself, in the dark, without pelvic thrust or body movement. In addition the bat's organ, like a snake's body poised to strike, pivots from its base. Male bats hang in there heroically, since Mother Nature decrees they do it upside down, hanging by their toes.

Far more accessible to survey is the two-foot-long penis of a rhinoceros. But if a female rhino looks as if the bottom has fallen out, do sympathize; Robert A. Wallace relates in his book *How They Do It:* during the hour or so the two-ton male stays mounted on her, his four legs swing free of the ground.

Some other hardy penile vistas include the ten-foot-long, foot-wide sex organ of the humpback (to be expected) male whale, and the overwhelmed armadillo, whose erect penis extends one third the length of his body. Also not to be overlooked is the penis of the pig—a foot and a half long and similar in appearance and action to a corkscrew. When thrust into a vagina, the penis's tip rotates deeper and deeper until it reaches the cervix. The pig's penetration is so deep that he ejaculates directly into the uterus, where he deposits a half-*quart* of semen (the average human male's ejaculation is a conservative teaspoonful). Though the dolphin also has a large muscular organ, he uses only the tip of it. This tip is attached to a "swivel" that enables him to use his small tool to rotate independently into the vagina. In courtship the dolphin is more generous (ah, yes!), for then he gratuitously inserts his large fin into her vagina.

The bull's large sex organ is easily identifiable once you know that it is S-shaped until it flaps into action, at which time it elongates and becomes exceedingly red. Since the bull's physique, says Wallace, does not allow for much swelling in the genital area, his organ's flagrant coloration might be caused by its never getting upright during a mating session.

Alas and alack, the King Kong of the jungle, the male gorilla, has a penis only two inches long, and the porcupine is another that has been hornswoggled—especially when you consider he needs, like anyone else, all the distance he can get from the female's spiny coat.

The watery world contains two of this globe's most unearthly penises. Take the male turtle: during erection his penis turns inside out, which could be the explanation for his wailing so loudly while doing it. And even more outlandish is the independent action of the penis of an octopus. In some species, the octopus's penis resides in one of his eight arms until it detaches itself to go solo in search of a vagina. This swimming sperm-laden penis/arm enters, copulates, and dies but continues to dangle from the female. Those nine-armed octopi are all females wandering around in a state of shock.

Even weirder is the penis of the flea; it comes in two sections, one thick, one thin. The thicker section slithers around, searching out a female flea's vagina, then turns, giving the skinny one privilege of entrance and visitation.

Unfortunately not having a hard time of it are some males, like the aforementioned octopi, who are born minus a penis. Among those that come a cropper are the toad, lobster, spider (who, like the octopus, uses one of his eight arms for copulation), many species of birds, and one species of the reptile family, the tuatara (*sphenodon punctatum*). The male seahorse also lacks a penis; the female has it. The inquisitive, penisless tick uses his nose. Far more fortunate are an enviable species of males, lizards and snakes, both of which have a dual set of functioning penises. Females of this species have been known to quake, since both organs are barbed and the males do it using both, one at a time.

Of course, never one to be put down is the human penis with its own unique specimens. In recent times two humans have been recorded as being born with a pair of penises plus an additional set of testicles. And, while it may get congested at times—such as during an erection—there is no evidence that these men were unhappy or maladjusted individuals.

Still another unique human penis surfaced only recently in the Soviet Union. During his imprisonment in a labor camp in Kharkov in the late 1960s, the Russian psychiatrist and sex therapist Dr. Mikhail Stern discovered an autosexual, a man whose penis was both flexible and rigid enough that he could insert it into his own anus and, by contracting his anal sphincter and his groin and buttocks muscles, bring himself to orgasm.

The autosexual is described by Dr. Stern as one (of which there are several in various labor camps throughout Russia, and no doubt more throughout the world) who is attracted to neither sex. His narcissism is so complete that he gets erotically aroused, even to the point of orgasm, just viewing his own bare body. Stern further describes the autosexual as "virtually autistic; he says very little, or nothing at all, and he rarely seeks out the company of his fellow inmates. He lives in absolute solitude but never seems affected by his loneliness." Not too shocking is Dr. Stern's report that photos of the autosexual, doing his solo act, are a popular form of pornography among prison inmates.

But the most influential penis of them all, from prehistoric to modern times, is the phallic symbol. The penis symbol, as an influence on human behavior, goes far back. Some historians claim that cave paintings from the Stone Age (28,000 to 22,000 B.C.) in southern France depict prehistoric man's spiritual dependency on the male sex symbol. Others claim this influence came much later, in the Neolithic era (around 10,000 B.C.), when the first shepherds probably made the mind-spinning discovery that doing it resulted in reproduction. Presumably this connection was not made until shepherds observed that a group of females in heat without a male had no babes. This blasting revelation—that a single male had the power to impregnate many females and so increase the herd—was the origin of phallic worship. From that moment on, penis was god.

From the Bronze Age in Corsica came solid evidence of the thrust of the penile symbol in prehistoric society. Archaeologists have unearthed on this rocky island several phallic stone monuments, some of which extend ten feet in height. Though these primitive pillars can hardly compete with the grandiose penile symbols of today—the Washington Monument, the Empire State Building, and the Eiffel Tower—they remain majestic symbols of achievement and devotion, especially when one recalls that prehistoric man had just begun to use a handy new building technique—leverage.

Later, in ancient Egypt's more sophisticated culture, the religious idol of a powerful deity was often enhanced with an oversized penis or dual sets of sex organs. Osiris was often depicted as a fiery bull with a triple penis (that's a lot of bull!) painted a challenging red. Even more blatant was a six-foot-high penis paraded through the streets of Alexandria by the king Ptolemy Philadelphus (now you know where "Philly" originated), who played it safe by funding the first translation of the Old Testament into Greek.

About the same time, across the globe, certain ancient Indian cults began parading penis puppets mounted on strings—doing their thing—during religious festivities. But the most active of all were the sixteen thousand wives in the harem of Krishna who used this god's sacred penile image as a religious dildo. Fanatics claimed this was a display of *deep* consecration. Realists snickered, claiming it was a boring necessity.

Ancient Judaic societies also poked around with displays of penile worship. One, a delicate touch, the other, a ball-busting display. First were touching males who, while giving an oath, placed their hands upon the testes of another (the origin of the word *testimony*). The ball-buster is that historians, who decipher primitive symbols, claim the Star of David is a prehistoric sign (two interlocked triangles, one

17

inverted) representing the male and female eternally doing it.

The ancient Greeks tagged the penis a phallus (also they coined the term for the clitoris, but that's another story). The Greeks were so hypnotized by the phallus that they deified it as a god potent enough to defy the "evil eye." This powerhouse was the god Priapus (today the source of priapism, a stuffy term for a disease that causes constant and painful erection of the penis), who extracted for his favors the sacrifice of an ass or a non-Greek male, both spitting images for lechery.

Before long the macho Romans, who were really hooked on gods—no fewer than thirty thousand deities were glorified by pagan Rome—succumbed to the hypnotic powers of the phallus. Dedicated to the spirit of expansion, the Romans required the propulsion of several phallic idols. One, the god Liber, projected his powers into every nook, and a few crannies, all over Rome. This deity's phallic image was plastered on the armor and chariots of conquering heroes; both males and females wore phallic jewelry to increase their sexual prowess; bakers made penis-shaped cookies and cakes in response to the belief that eating the symbol of a god made one doubly blessed (a pseudocannibalism that prevails); phallic images adorned the private altars of most Roman homes and, in gardens, protected plants and flowers. (Yes, it is difficult to conceive the penis as the first bobbing scarecrow. Or vice versa.) Naturally, shopkeepers placed the phallic image over doorways to bring added cash flow, and civic leaders dangled it from town gates and walls to repel disease and invasion. And the great poets of Rome treated the phallic god like the rock star he was, exalting his racy look and sexy powers in poems, ditties, and tunes.

Centuries later, in disgust and revolt, the Christian theologian Augustine quoted the Roman historian Varro's description of the powerful persuasion of the phallic god. To ward off the evil eye, you might give it a glance:

> . . the rites of Liber were celebrated . . . so immodestly and licentiously that . . . the male genitals were worshipped in honour of the god—and this not with any modest secrecy but with open and exulting depravity. That shameful part of the body was . . . placed with great pomp on wagons and carried about to the crossroads in the country, and at last into the city . . . a whole month was dedicated to Liber. During it, all the citizens used the most disgraceful words until the Phallus . . . had been put to rest again. It was necessary that the most honourable of the matrons should publicly place a wreath on that disgraceful effigy. The god Liber had to be propitiated to ensure the future of the crops, and the evil eye had to be repelled from the fields by compelling a married woman to do in public that which not even a harlot might do under the eyes of married women in the theatre.

Best to leave the sacrifices of these married ladies for another story and, instead, reveal those performed as a public service by Roman virgins before their wedding day—the breaking of their hymens on the rigid phallic image of the deity Mutunus Tutunus as a previewing audience cheered them on.

There seemed no end to the penetration of the phallic symbol, at least not until the Christians took their turn with this ball, and then, like Rome, the phallus tumbled. True, there were sightings of a phallic idol as late as the eighteenth century in Naples, but, tragic to tell, the penis was in Christian drag and baptized the Great Toe of Saint Cosmo.

In the twentieth century the phallus rose again! A travesty of its former image, of course, since science is now the top banana for this ball, and Freud, in his resurrection, made the phallus sublimely subliminal!

3

MANUAL POLLUTION AND THE "BIG M" PLAGUE

Though Christians deflated the phallic symbol as a god, the penis as a personal object remained a sacred entity. God or no, Christian or not, no one was allowed to fool around with the penis. Especially not its keeper. As an evil act, self-masturbation has a sustained history dating back to ancient times. The term originated in Rome as *manusturbo*, meaning "to defile (or disturb) with the hands." Romans associated masturbation with the evil left hand (what the right hand was doing was a sacrilege!) and the Latin word for left is *sinister*. And sinister are the numerous English terms used for centuries, even to this day, as euphemisms for penile self-stimulation.

Take your hands from your pockets and come to grips with some of these: abuse oneself, ball off, box the Jesuit and get cockroaches, bring down by hand, choke the chicken, come one's mutton, diddle, do-it-yourself, express a secret vice, fight one's turkey, fist-fuck, gallop one's antelope, gallop one's maggot, get one's nuts off, five against one, flog one's sausage, fondle one's fig, and frig.

Take a deep breath. Now: grind away, hand job, hotrod, jack off, jag off, jazz oneself, jerk off, jerk one's gherkin, keep the census down, Levy and Frank, manipulate one's mango, manual pollution, manstrupration, means of weakness and debility, mount a corporal and four, onanism, Portuguese pump, pound one's pomegranate, pull one's pud, pump one's pickle, pump one's python, rub-up, screw off, secret vice, self-infanticide, sling one's jelly, snap the rubber, solitary sin, squeeze the lemon, stroke the lizard, take oneself in hand, whack off, whip one's wire, and yank one's star.

Of course there are hundreds, if not thousands, more. In his *Slang and Euphemism*, Richard A. Spears gives a stimulating list; indeed most of the above appear there. Some handy advice though: Spears euphemistically itemizes his masturbatory list under the heading Waste Time.

Historically, masturbation is a dry subject. Consider the ancient Greeks, who, though living in an erotic culture, thought masturbation was, at best, something you did when you had nothing else going for you. Islamic civilizations deemed it okay, *but* only in a rare emergency. The most self-serving were the ancient Chinese and Indians, who said, "do it but keep it dry," for *any* loss of semen was considered wasting and wasteful since its replacement could only come from a female's vaginal juices. But the Talmud is heavy-handed; it forbids Jews to hold their penises while urinating *unless* their wives are immediately available for intercourse.

Even the Pyramid Texts from ancient Egypt considered

masturbation a pain in the ass. These sacred tomes describe the offshoot of a male god's masturbation as procreation with delivery through the anus. Now that *is* playing dirty.

Still, until the fourth century A.D. masturbation was entertained by most cultures in the world as a necessary evil. For example, during wartime it was tagged a soldier's joy. But all this changed when Europe, with the fall of the Roman Empire and the Classical Age, blew a fuse and entered the Dark Ages until the eleventh century.

This blackout—the decay of urban life, advanced learning, and literacy—was conducive to sitting around in the dark of ignorance and telling horror stories of hell and damnation. Then came the sixth century, when going to hell in a handsling became a big possibility, and the Western Church's publication of a set of codes, the Penitentials, which defined and prescribed penances for all sins. Near the top of the list, for serious sinning, was masturbation, specifically defined and handily described in twenty-five detailed paragraphs. Indeed the codes not only provided a handbook for how to do it, but listed who was doing it and what the cost would be for handling.

Penances were broken down by age, marital and religious status (the clergy were definitely not excluded), and extended from one day (youths with greenhorns) to three years (pulsating bishops). But, considering hell's fires, these penances were seldom heavy, although time consuming. They were usually spiritual chores such as singing psalms, going on pilgrimages, saying prayers, and fasting. However, the fasting was nothing serious, for even the worst penitent was allowed bread and water.

For centuries the Western Church had fought—but lost —its battle against "the monstrous act" of self-masturbation. The seventeenth century brought the Age of Rationalization, when the movers and the shakers shifted from the clergy to men of science and philosophy.

Previously the Church had used sin and the fear of damnation for its powerhouse. Science switched this fear to sickness, insanity, and death. One of the first to discover this new scourge was a Lausanne, Switzerland, physician, S. A. Tissot, who described it in his book, *On Onanism or a physical dissertation on the ills produced by masturbation*. The symptoms of this illness included cloudiness of ideas; pimples on the face, thighs, and breast; blisters on the nose; painful itching; constipation; hemorrhoids; and eventually, decay of bodily powers; madness; consumption; tumors of the bladder; painful permanent erection; and (the good news) numbness.

Tissot said these ills could be contracted one at a time, several together, or for a lucky few, none at all.

Until the Age of Reason, masturbation had been condemned solely on moral grounds. What would suddenly cause a moral issue to become a multifaceted disease capable of destroying physical and mental health? One recent theory is that syphilis, which had reached epidemic proportions in Europe during the sixteenth century, was the real culprit. Religious and social stigma made patients ashamed to reveal their sleeping around. As a result physicians concluded that syphilis came from the "solitary disease."

By 1810 physicians throughout Central Europe, France, and Britain were warning self-abusers of early death, malformed children, epilepsy, insanity, impotency, frigidity, tuberculosis, and paralysis. The only treatment the medical profession offered the chronic abuser was cutting the nerves to the penis and painful cauterization of the prostate gland. This "cure" drove many to suicide, and the rest suffered certain impotency.

The "in-hand" was out of hand. Patients began dropping like flies. The Big M plague was so devastating that physicians stopped prescribing such lightweight cures as cold baths, strenuous exercise, swimming, opiates, quinine, lupulin, potassium bromate, cannabis, or camphor.

Religious condemnation, jail sentences, commitment to

mental institutions had all failed. And, finally, even medical science could not save those lost to "the monstrous act."

At last, in 1818 a medical breakthrough came. The solution—French underwear—was discovered by a famous orthopedic surgeon, G. Jalade-Lafond. He claimed the "immoderate release of spermic fluid" could be controlled if the abuser would wear his penis corset (which went from the shoulders to the top of the knees!). This device intrigued everyone except the Germans, who were positive the cause of masturbation was "French influences." So entrenched was this belief that a German physician wrote a book in which he claimed that the ultimate antidote for masturbation would be a resurgence of German nationalism. A cure that would exclude, obviously, saving self-molesting British, Poles, Italians, and others. But apparently German patriotism was not the equal of the Big M plague, for in 1829 a German physician, Dr. Johann Fleck, introduced a variant invention for prevention: Teutonic-style underwear.

Dr. Fleck described his invention in a book titled *The Erroneous Turns of the Sex Drive*. The abuser/patient was zapped into a leather vest (laced securely up the back for additional security) which had attached leather garters from which hung a metal tube that held the penis. The tube had a convenient tiny aperture at the end to facilitate elimination. But Dr. Fleck did not know all the erroneous turns of the sex-driven, for practicers of "the evil habit" were soon snapping their leather garters and dropping their tubes.

In 1831 a Munich surgical instrument maker retailored the vest by adding a steel belt from which *steel* garters and a steel penis tube dangled and all of which were surrounded by a steel shield. After a successful experiment on a thirteen-year-old boy, he said, "I feel happy to have contributed my share to combating this pernicious evil." There is no quote from the boy (other than the clanging of his underwear).

In 1848 the British made their contribution to saving

mankind from itself. Their device was much the same as the 1831 German model except there were two metal penis tubes: one for the penis to just hang in there, the other the patient used, by pushing his penis sideways, when he wanted to urinate. The British, with their sense of fair play, also created the first device to save "the corrupt woman."

But British medical science made a much greater discovery about this time—a new strain in the Big M disease—spermatorrhea or sexual neurasthenia.

British author Charles Drysdale described a victim of spermatorrhea as one "who wakes suddenly from a stupor, just as the discharge is pouring out, which he will try in vain to check; or perhaps he will not wake till it's over, and then as lethargic consciousness, which of itself tells him what has taken place, slowly awakens, he puts down his hand and sickens with despair, as he perceives the fatal drain, and thinks on the gloomy morrow which will follow."

What caused the Big M, after it crossed the English Channel, to strike only "stuporous victims"? The "disease" was the same but the patient had changed. The British considered males on the European Continent so base they would allow themselves consciousness during such debasing action, but never the Victorian gentleman.

Haplessly, the Victorian schoolboy was often less than stuporous. The English physician and Victorian sex authority William Acton described the boy who masturbated as one of a "frame stunted and weak, the muscles underdeveloped, the eye is sunken and heavy, the complexion is sallow, pasty or skin moist. The boy shuns the society of others, creeps about alone, joins with repugnance in the amusements of his schoolfellows. He cannot look anyone in the face, and becomes sluggish and enfeebled, and if his evil habits are persisted in, he may end becoming a drivelling idiot or peevish valetudinarian. Such boys are seen in all stages of degeneration," etc., etc., etc.

How this poor nebbie had the strength to masturbate is never explained.

As a youth in late Victorian England, Havelock Ellis says he was so fearful of becoming a victim of spermatorrhea he had "reached the conclusion that there was no outcome except by death or possibly becoming a monk."

In Germany, in 1886, Richard Freiherr von Krafft-Ebing published the first of his many books on *Psychopathia Sexualis* in which he claimed childhood masturbation was the cause of perversion and many adult sadistic crimes, including *murder*. These books, although medical textbooks with the sexier parts written in Latin, became bestsellers in many countries and were popular for almost eight decades (the last edition was printed in 1965 in the United States). Krafft-Ebing made a mint, for his books were filled with gory—but actual—tales that excited, disgusted, terrified, and delighted.

The Big M plague had crossed the Atlantic and leveled the puritanical Yanks in the 1830s. Sylvester Graham, a self-made nutritionist and the inventor of the graham cracker, proclaimed that all of the abovementioned ills and more awaited those who misused their sexual organs. He claimed that orgasm, with the loss of an ounce of semen, was equivalent to the loss of several ounces of blood. Therefore, *every* ejaculation was a nail in the male's coffin. His solution for a healthy mind and body was to limit sex to not more than twelve times a year and that to be strung out and only with your wife. To cut down on sexual desire he further advocated the use of hard mattresses, cold showers, a diet that included large amounts of hominy, rye meal, and unbolted flour from which the American delicacy—his graham cracker—was made.

Another champion of dry penises and dry cereals was the inventor of cornflakes, John Harvey Kellogg. He claimed masturbation was more dangerous than sodomy, for there were no "bounds to its indulgence." He, though, made no dietary suggestions for self-abusers, for he believed those addicted were averse to simple foods—not to mention girls and piety.

Then in the 1860s, the founder of U.S. pediatrics, Dr. Abraham Jacobi, claimed infantile paralysis was caused by self-abuse.

But corsets, vests, shields, metal tubes, handcuffs (applied at night and behind the back), and diets were all put aside when the "perfect" product burst into the neighborhood drugstores of Europe and the United States. The device was simple, small, cheap, and—best of all—*immediately* effective. It was a small metal ring lined with spikes. Some had bows tied on, but they were just a jaunty touch to attract the jaded eye. A prominent British surgeon wrote raves about it, saying one must "see the effects of this little instrument to see its value."

Other instruments, machines, and devices tried to replace it, claiming theirs to be a better mousetrap; in fact, between 1856 and 1932 the U.S. Patent Office granted thirty-three patents to inventors of sexual restraints, each complex. One example is the invention by a Miss Perkins, a nurse—not a patient—in a mental hospital. This consisted of a leather-lined suit of steel armor plating with holes for urinating and a padlocked rear trapdoor for defecating. An attendant with a key was, oddly, not recommended.

In the early twentieth century, Sigmund Freud said the traditional education of the young was as realistic as sending people on a polar expedition dressed in summer clothing and equipped with a map of the Italian lakes. Sex education was not specified by Freud, for it was nonexistent, even to the medical profession. But Freud and Havelock Ellis waded into this icy, barren land and gave birth to a new science—sexology.

Theologians and medical scientists had done their best

for two thousand years to take sex to the laundry. It was now time to hang out the wash.

The next one to appear on the human-sex-reform scene was a zoologist, Dr. Alfred C. Kinsey, renowned for his collection and classification of insects. Leave it to Middlesville, U.S.A. (Bloomington, Indiana), to have a zoologist conducting a university class on marriage. For Kinsey's ignorance of his subject and that of those he was to instruct led to the creation of an institute that would eventually contain the second largest collection of sexual material in the world. The first, allegedly, is the Vatican Library in Rome, which has been collecting it to save the world from vice.

And so the next hotbed for a sexual breakthrough would be a town appropriately named Bloomington? True, the time was 1938, and soon most of Europe and parts of Asia and Africa would be busy blowing holes in each other. Still, that a fresh approach to sexual problems came from Corn Country, U.S.A., in the middle of the Bible Belt, does blow minds.

What started it all was Kinsey's reply, during a rap session at a fraternity, to questions on whether masturbation, petting, and homosexuality were harmful. "Neither I nor anyone else knows the answer to many of these questions because of our lack of knowledge, but if you and many like you will be willing to contribute your sexual histories, I will be able, eventually, to answer at least some of these questions." And the answer given to that humble statement has resulted in over eighteen thousand direct-interview case histories, now stored in the Kinsey Institute archives.

And who was the slap-happiest at keeping it up with the Joneses? Kinsey says the adolescent male, whose maximum frequency of masturbation is two to three per day. And eighty-eight percent of sixteen- to twenty-year-olds actively masturbate. At fifteen years of age, the frequency of masturbation (comparing the highest individual ratings) is 2.5 times that of a thirty-year-old and four times that of a fifty-year-old.

Ultimately, ninety-two percent of all U.S. males will masturbate to orgasm (and the statistics from Europe come close to that figure). But a college education (or even the prospect of one!) will increase the action to ninety-six percent and the frequency will also rise.

In the working world the high achiever for frequency is the professional male (especially if an inactive Protestant) who does it twice as often as the laborer. But still the overall high achiever is that adolescent working away at his two or three per day. No wonder the teens are considered at an awkward age—it's a marvel they have the strength to walk.

Those who don't—or won't—cut the mustard are a mixed bag: some try self-masturbation and turn off; some are busy with others sexually; and some are faithful to the teachings from their schul or church (orthodox Jews are *very* low achievers and devout Roman Catholics run a close second).

Shere Hite, in *The Hite Report on Male Sexuality* published in 1981, says that ninety percent of the more than seven thousand men she interviewed enjoyed masturbation and that eighty-four percent do it for an orgasm. She found, "Most men feel guilty and inadequate about masturbating, at the same time they enjoy it tremendously . . . and seemed to have a great sense of freedom and fun while doing it . . . to experiment . . . to simply play around and have a good time with their bodies. *Almost no men told anyone else that they did this.*" (Emphasis ours.)

The human male is of two ilks about observing himself during self-eroticism. From Kinsey we learn that some of the most vigorous heterosexual males avoid any observation, preferring to do it in the dark while focusing inwardly on a fantasy. Yet there are many others who prefer the opposite. Hite found that eighty-two percent prefer the traditional hand manipulation and the other eight percent rubbing against some smooth object.

A Kinsey statistic says that the average male takes two

minutes to masturbate, while others can vary between ten seconds and an hour or more.

There are also some human males who attempt self-fellatio—unfortunately only two or three in a thousand can pull it off. Again, those in the awkward age of adolescence top the list. Also flexible enough outside of the human species are some mammals such as goats, cats, dogs, mandrills, chimps, rhesus monkeys, macaques, and other primates.

In the animal kingdom, masturbation has been observed in male camels, sheep, parrots, elephants, ponies, bears, goats, apes, stags, cats, horses, bulls, peewits, dogs, porcupines, and dolphins.

Research in animal masturbation is seldom boring, for each of the above brings its own style and technique. Goats are flexible—they can stimulate their penises with their forelegs (one at a time, of course), or, if they prefer, autofellate themselves to orgasm. Porcupines use a stick, accurately. Welsh ponies do it with their eyes closed, yet they are wide-eyed during mating. Stags do it by rubbing against trees—not their penises, their antlers! A heady experience to be sure. Sheep and camels do it by pressing down on anything that is handy. And elephants do it by tucking their four- to five-foot penises between their hind legs. Bears do the same but only—supposedly—while watching other bears mate. Gorillas "reportedly" do it only in captivity—while other species of apes do it anywhere. Dogs do it by rubbing against you, autofellatio, and licking their nipples. Some cats do the same, although less overtly. The show-off dolphin has done it for applause from the grandstand in marine parks.

Another Kinsey statistic says that twenty-six to twenty-eight percent of U.S. males have masturbated animals while masturbating themselves. If twenty-eight percent seems an inflated statistic, you live in an urban area. For Kinsey found that the percentage could go as high as sixty-five percent in some areas of the Western United States. The frequency of sexual contacts between participating human males and animals varied from once or twice in a lifetime to eight times per week, and the time span for ongoing relationships ranged from two or three years up to fifteen. Kinsey also found that this type of masturbation was more prevalent with preadolescent and adolescent boys (they're at it again?) in rural areas. Also, "loners" in the Western United States were high on this list.

Probably seventy-two percent of the urban males in the Eastern United States are shaking their heads, wondering what the attraction is. Kinsey says for young 'uns it's curiosity and comparison study, while for those over and on the hill it is expediency and something called "habitual indulgence."

And Kinsey adds that fidelity, when given, is not one-sided—there are "records of male dogs who forsake the female of their own species in preference for sexual contact that might be had with a human partner."

4

EROGENY—A BEGINNING TO MAKE BOTH ENDS MEET

Yankee Doodle keep it up
Yankee doodle dandy.
Mind the music and the step,
And with the girls be handy.

This ditty's tuneful advice, by Anonymous in the eighteenth century, could also apply to the handy maneuvers used by many males whose sex organs are bent for doing it.

In the human animal these maneuvers are called foreplay, which in the recent past was called petting. Today this euphemism has bottomed out, along with spooning, larking, and courting. And, in some areas of the United States petting has escalated, literally and figuratively, to screwing, which is a euphemism for balling, which is a euphemism for fucking.

Fucking, by the way, needs all the euphemisms it can get. According to Eric Partridge in *Origins:* "Fuck shares with cunt two distinctions: they are the only two Slang English words excluded from all general and etymological dictionaries since the 18th Century and the only two . . . outside of medical and other semi-official reports and learned papers, that still could not be printed anywhere within the British Commonwealth of Nations until late 1961."

In the first half of the twentieth century petting was what heterosexual Yankee males did to females so innocent they thought Fucking was somewhere in interior China. In the last few decades since the sexual revolution most female Yanks know, and enjoy, the latitude of Fucking and have hopes for the longitude.

As living things ascend the evolutionary ladder, petting plays an increasing part in courtship. In the lower orders, erogenous zones are meager, if at all, and sexual excitement and sexual intercourse are preprogrammed and periodic. Indeed, on the bottom rung of the evolutionary ladder are several species of marine life who do it sexually not at all. Such include sponges, oysters, jellyfish, corals, and other lie-a-beds. Higher up in the animal kingdom the female usually has to be in heat and the male in rut. But on his top rung of this evolutionary ladder, the human male is far from in a rut. From head to toe, minus shell, feathers, thick hide, or much fur, the human male sports a throbbing, quivering mass of erogenous zones that after puberty function twenty-four hours a day and 365¼ days a year.

In the rest of the animal kingdom, sex is a *very* hard sell unless the female is in heat. And the heated season could be a torrid, beastly fling limited to two weeks out of a year. Because the male animal is ready and up for longer periods, he nudges around a lot in an attempt to rush the heating season. And though it seldom gets him entry to the inner circle, the male animal continues to playfully nip, surrep-

titiously mount, tug away at hide, or drag on fur. Some fer-
vids even stoop to urinating on their chosen ones.

Actually, it is difficult to observe most animals in the
sexual act (other than domestic breeds who feel right at
home), as many seem to prefer privacy and a place of their
own. It has been suggested this penchant for privacy is a
built-in safety device because, during mating, the attention
of the participants is directed away from potential predators
and rivals.

Also these participants in animal foreplay, as with humans, do not confine their pawing and clawing to members
of the opposite sex. In *Sexual Behavior of the Human Female*,
Kinsey says that the male baboon, lion, porpoise, porcupine,
and monkey "have been known to have exclusive but temporary sexual desire for their own sex."

But not so temporary are the lusts of an odd species of
bedbug (thought they were all alike, did you?) which is
equipped with a penis and an additional sex organ reserved
to receive the semen from another male bedbug. This accommodating bedbug then ejaculates his sperm and that of
his recent male sex partner into a female bedbug, who certainly gets more than she bargained for.

The male octopus is physically irresistible, for he greets
the female with one slap after another with his eight arms,
then uses one and all to squeeze and envelope her. Whales
are more considerate; they hug and rub with their flippers.
Rabbits visually excite each other by checking out their
white underbellies—then he, the sneak before his leap, urinates on her. Penguins take foreplay very seriously, for they
nod and nod and nod and nod at each other, and then com-
mences an exchange of interminable yapping. Prairie dogs,
sea lions, and chimps nuzzle and kiss. So do elephants, but
the male does it French style with his trunk in her mouth.
Gorillas nip, hug, grab, and fondle all the areas humans usually do. But the hair on the head, shoulders, and arms of

the male chimpanzee stands on end to tell a gal she turns him on.

The male porcupine, with his body only a mother could love, whines a wily ditty in a high falsetto voice to attract his spiny damsel. Before she runs away, thinking he's gone off half-cocked (remember, he has a tiny penis), he rears up on his hind legs and prances forward, baldly pointing his erect penis. As Ms. porcupine warily eyes this flasher he urinates on her from the safe but trigger-happy distance of six or more feet. If she is in heat she sticks it out, otherwise she runs like hell, leaving him to hold his sack.

With his bigger brain and vivid imagination, the human male first gets erotic arousal from a variety of mind games. Kinsey claims males achieve arousal from thirty-three psychosexual experiences. These mental and visual stimuli are the same for heterosexual and homosexual males and none of them are, statistically, electrifying. They include looking at pornography, burlesque shows, genitals (including their own), animals doing it, and erotic art forms. Also listed is reading erotic writing and sexual graffiti, especially in johns. Fantasizing about past and future sex partners and voyeurism are other stimuli used by male humans.

Kinsey says females are less influenced by these experiences. For them erotic arousal is usually stimulated by direct physical contact. Kinsey goes on to say, "Many females are surprised anyone finds the observation of male genitalia erotically stimulating . . . many consider [the male organ] ugly and repulsive in appearance . . . and the sight of it may actually inhibit their erotic responses." This sentence was published in 1953. After thirty years and a sexual revolution one wonders if the penis is still such an ugly duckling.

After erotic mental or visual stimulation takes place, most males take immediate action to get reaction. For openers come groping and pawing; then, a close second, kissing—but not all over, at least not all over the world.

'Tis said Jonathan Swift, in a snit, one day asked, "Lord, I wonder what fool it was that first invented kissing." An answer to this query could be Havelock Ellis's solution two centuries later. Ellis claimed this invention—with sly intentions—originated from the palpitations of the antennae of insects and snails and the caressing birds do with their bills. The tactile kiss, Ellis tells us, is generally known in mammals. And in humans it is both ancient and primitive and possibly related to a mother's licking her young, thus a manifestation of a fundamental animal impulse. Also the impulse to bite lies in the origin of kissing, since many male animals grasp the female with their teeth during sexual intercourse. But the kiss, for affectionate use, is not to everyone's taste. Ellis explains in *Studies in the Psychology of Sex:*

> The kiss thus understood is not very widely spread and is not usually found among rude and uncultured peoples. We can trace it in Aryan and Semitic antiquity, but in no very pronounced form; Homer scarcely knew it, and the Greek poets seldom mention it. Today it may be said to be known all over Europe except in Lapland. Even in Europe it is probably a comparatively modern discovery . . . Throughout eastern Asia it is unknown; thus in Japanese literature kisses and embraces have no existence. Among nearly all of the black races of Africa lovers never kiss nor do mothers usually kiss their babies . . . Among the American Indians the tactile kiss is, for the most part, unknown . . . however . . . in many parts of the world . . . it still exists between a mother and her baby, and this seems to support the view . . . that the lovers' kiss is developed from the maternal kiss.

Ellis goes on to say that the kiss, as an expression of sexual love, was unknown during medieval times in Europe except in the more cultivated classes. Also, the kiss in the Near East was largely monopolized for sacred uses, and Romans used it more for reverence and respect than as a method for sexual excitement. Among the early Christians the kiss had a sacramental significance reserved for the relics of saints and the foot of the pope (a practice which began in the eighth century when a pope cut off one of his hands after, supposedly, becoming unnerved when a woman squeezed his hand while kissing it).

Ellis claims the olfactory kiss is used in more parts of the world, especially in China. It has three phases:

> (1) the nose is applied to the cheek of the beloved person; (2) there is a long nasal inspiration accompanied by lowering the eyelids; (3) there is a slight smacking of the lips without the application of the mouth to the embraced cheek . . . the whole process . . . is founded on sexual desire and the desire for food, smell being the same sense employed in both fields.

The Chinese find the European kiss odious. It suggests voracious cannibals, and Ellis tells us that mothers frighten their children by threatening to give them "the white man's kiss."

Kissing is an art. *The Perfumed Garden*, an ancient poetic how-to book, describes how mouth-to-mouth kissing for erotic stimulation is done:

> The kiss should be sonorous: it originates with the tongue touching the palate, lubricated by saliva. It is produced by the movement of the tongue in the mouth and by the displacement of the saliva, provoked by the suction. The kiss given to the superficial outer part of the lips, and making a noise comparable to the one by which you call your cat, gives no pleasure.

In the twentieth century *The Sensuous Man* tells us how to practice kissing before nibbling at delicate erogenous areas other than the mouth of a sexual partner:

Place a small grape in your mouth. Keeping it between your teeth and your tongue, rotate it with your tongue. Be extremely careful not to break the skin of the grape. Roll it from side to side in your mouth and knead it with your lips. When you are able to manipulate the grape in this fashion without rupturing the skin, then you are applying approximately the correct amount of pressure necessary to stimulate and excite her nipples without causing any pain to these very sensitive erogenous zones. If you are able to bring the grape to orgasm so much the better.

The next phase of seduction is the choice between one and 1001 postures to take in preparation for entering. Most males do this the hard way.

About ten million years ago, as man slowly evolved from the primates, this was never a problem. There was only one position a male could take for rear entry of the female while she was on all fours facing her fate alone. Then, as humans stood erect, the female's vagina, visibly, did a disappearing act. This took many, many centuries; therefore males had ample time to research another approach. Thus frontal copulation became the second position and a new sexual vista emerged when two faces—in addition to two genitals—were brought together. One can safely assume that personal identification during such intense intimacy was the birth of the sensual experience.

The first illustrated *and* written description of various sexual positions came from the Chinese in the second century B.C. There were only thirty. In the first century B.C. the Roman poet Ovid wrote *Ars Amatoria,* in which he described in detail how a Roman woman positions herself for doing it. So descriptive was Ovid, he is said to be the only genius to take up pornography. The first true sex manual came in 300 A.D. in India, Vatsyayana's *Kama Sutra.* This poetic guide to sexual enjoyment lists eighty-four positions. The scoreboard quickly changed after this, when a commentator on the

Kama Sutra came up with 729 postures. The last countdown, 1,001, came from an eye-tearing twentieth-century porno book, *One Thousand and One Sexual Embraces* (anonymous).

Among its eighty-four positions, the *Kama Sutra* has a few that require penetrating inspection. One, the "Supportive Position," depicts the female leaping onto the back of a standing male. She then quickly flings her right leg over his right shoulder. As she clasps her ankle with her right hand, she swings both hips around to spear herself on his erect penis, leaving her left leg to dangle behind free of the floor. Both partners are gazing left, in awe, at her outstretched arm as she balances in her left hand a glass filled with wine.

Another, the "Spinning Top Position," has two variations. The more acrobatic shows the male doing a full back bend with the female perched on top of his erect penis. She is reaching back to grasp her cocked left thigh with her left hand. She is using her right arm and leg to propel herself around and around and around his penis. Her gaze remains riveted on the sole of her cocked left foot. His gaze is directed heavenward.

The second variation has the male seated in a semi-reclining position with the female perched both on his lower stomach and his erect penis. His left leg is doubled back with the sole of his foot propelling her around and around his penis. To keep her legs out of the way she has tossed the right one over her right shoulder, with the toes pointed skyward. Her left leg is bent and tucked, at the ankle, under her chin. She gazes at the toes of her left foot as she spins around the penis. His gaze is glazed.

The "Fixing a Nail" position portrays a male kneeling, facing due west. His outstretched arms are supporting the torso of a female crouched on one leg pointing west. Her head is faced to the south but her breasts are dangling southeast. For symmetry her opposite leg is bent backward so she can tuck her toes behind an earlobe.

The ancient Chinese had a sexual health manual,

Goddess of the Shell, which prescribed eight postures for therapeutic lovemaking. Eight medicinal benefits could be achieved by males who did the following:

1. To concentrate his semen, the male should, twice daily, penetrate a female who is facing him on her side. Each penetration is to cease after eighteen inner strokes of love. This must be done for a period of fifteen consecutive days.

2. To rest his spirit, a male should give twenty-seven strokes of love to his partner who is reclining while he kneels between her thighs. This should be done three times a day for twenty consecutive days.

3. For a male concerned with his internal organs, the prescription is thirty-six strokes of love, performed four times a day for twenty days. His partner is curled up in a ball on her side, and he is required to enter her from behind as he warms his stomach against her buttocks.

4. To strengthen his bones, both partners must curl into each other with the female's right leg outstretched and the left leg raised and bent. Forty-five inner strokes of love are needed five times a day for a period of ten days.

5. For increased blood circulation, the female switches the above leg positions and must be lying on her side. Six times a day he must give her fifty-four strokes and keep it up for twenty days.

6. Sixty-three strokes seven times daily for ten consecutive days will increase his blood supply. He must stretch out and *allow* dominance.

7. To increase his bone marrow is somewhat trickier, for the male must give, in a supine position, eight times daily, seventy-two inner strokes of love for *as many days as it takes* to receive a benefit.

8. Finally, to revitalize his whole being, the male must position the female so her bent legs support her buttocks as he enters her from a kneeling position. She must remain this

way till he gives her eighty-one strokes of love, nine times a day, nine days in succession.

Since male orgasm is not allowed in any of the above remedies, we can only assume this Chinaman is in better shape than he knows.

The *Kama Sutra* has more industrious activities than inner love strokes planned for the penis. This manual describes nine separate movements the male's penis should make during intercourse. From start to finish it goes something like this: First the penis moves forward into the vagina; once inside, it must turn and churn, guided by the male's hand; next the penis must strike, then stroke the upper part of the vagina; then do the same for the lower part; this is followed by several aggressive withdrawals and reentries of the vagina, as if to give it a blow; the rhythm then alters so the penis *slowly* rubs only one area at a time of the vagina; next the penis must press down very deep; and, finally, picking up the pace, both the penis and the vagina must alternately press toward each other, with mounting force, until both achieve a climax.

For the laid-back penis the *Kama Sutra* gives eight specific movements a sexual partner should do during oral sex. They are the obvious kissing, biting, rubbing, pressing, sucking, and swallowing. G. Legman, a delightful historian of erotica, took over three hundred pages to describe oral sex in his book *Ora-Genitalism*. Fortunately, he adds, oral sex is much easier to do than describe. A fair portion of the book is reserved for cunnilingus, but he does claim there are 14,288,400 positions for exciting the genitals with oral techniques—not all of which are defined.

For centuries man has been describing in words the act of copulation. While prose and poetry are certainly stimulating when they tackle genital unions, for a quickie the euphemism can't be beat. They are so varied, it is worth categorizing some of the more stirring ones.

CHORES

In the works
Give the business to
Lay some pipe
Plant the oats
To plug
Caulking
Haul one's ashes
Plugging away
Blanket drill
Fix the plumbing
Shaking the sheets
Churning it
Give a hosing
Mattress jigging
Chamber work
Make the chimney smoke
Smoke your pipe
Busy one's wick
Knock the stuffing out
Get laid

SINFUL AND BAD

An act of shame
Improper intercourse
Venereal act
Dirty work at the crossroads
Behind-the-door work
Carnal connection
Fornication
The ringing of Hell's bells

AUTOMOTIVE

Drive home
Cranking
Get one's oil fixed
Play garage
To service a station
A coupling
Go along for the ride
Zigging and zagging
Make a pass

HOLY AND GOOD

The act of Heaven
Nuptial rites
Consummation
Conjugal rites
Sacrifice to Venus
The act of generation

REASONABLE

To occupy
Break for lunch
The use of sex
Get on board
What mother did before me
Fit end to end
Join paunches
Both ends supple
Crack it
Give a hole to hide in
Consensual act
Bim bam, thank you ma'am

MEDICINAL AND THERAPEUTIC

Playing doctor
Intercourse
Act of androgynation
Copulation
To have sex
Coitus
Horizontal exercise
Cure for the horn
Give me some skin
Flesh session
Sleep together

COMFORTS

Have it off
Belly warming
Act of kindness
Handy and dandy
A hot lay
Bit of hard for a bit of soft
Cool out
To get one's nuts cracked
A snug for a bit of stiff
Go soak yourself
Get one's rocks off

ENTERTAINING

Tail tickling
Joyride
Buzz the balls
Belly bumping

ENTERTAINING (cont'd.)

A toss in the hay
Bottoms up
Four-legged frolic
Twatting
A squeeze and a squirt
Frigging
Dickey dunking
Rumbusticate
Getting Jack in the orchard
Buttock stirring
Hanky-panky
Fucking
Play around
Turn a trick

HISTORICAL EVENTS

What Eve did to Adam
What Adam did to Eve
French connection
Waterloo
The first game ever played

SAD TO SAY

A screw-up
To qualify
Have one's will
Get a shove in one's blind
  eye
Make the scene
A cram
Get into her pants
Grumbling and a grunt

43

SAD TO SAY (cont'd.)

Scraping the bottom
Give one a stab
Take a turn on Shooting Hill
Shaft clubbing
A daub of the brush
Impale
Switch-hitting
Making out
Messing around
Shacking up
Give a poke

ROMANTIC

Making love
The sex embrace
Love's life
The act of darkness
Succeed amorously
A gallant act
The act of love
The acme of delight
A bit of black velvet
Hair courting
Play house

BIBLICAL

To know
Enter into

GOOD SPORTS

Shoot one's wad
Yo-yoing
Cocking
Irish whist
Horsemanship
Bouncey-bouncey
A turkey shoot
Getting it climbing
The splits
Send to the showers
Come about
Catch an oyster
A game in the cock loft
Heave anchor
Get some action
Get up and git
Do dice in the dark
Go all the way
Make a pass at
Doing it all the way

MUSICAL COMEDIES

Play your organ
Dance the meat polka
Jazzing it up
Jigging around
Thrumming
Ring your bell
Dance the buttock jig

THE DELI

Give juice for jelly
Lady feasting
Creamstick
Meat delivery
Picking cabbage
A hot pudding
Get one's oats
Porkbellies
Jam making
Curling greens
Mutton serving
Fish and dish
Honeypot of Venus
Hot roll with cream
Ground rations
Horizontal refreshment
Fruit that made man wise

THE DELI (cont'd.)

Hide the salami
A hunk of tail

REAL BORES

Trot out pussy
Be familiar with
Give standing room
Sleep with
Trading
Shack up with someone
Casual sex
Put out
Make out
Bag job
Get laid
Look at the ceiling over a
    shoulder

Nowhere is this listing the end all of it. For that one should research, till at least the first decade of the twentieth century, the philological erotica collection of physician Henry N. Cary reposited at the Kinsey Institute for Research. Dr. Cary listed twenty-nine pages of euphemisms for copulation. 'Tis rumored no one has read it through because it's a grind.

Whatever it's called, sexual intercourse in America is on the rise, and the Yankee penis is more popular than ever. Take the comparison between these two statistics. In 1953 Alfred Kinsey reported in *Sexual Behavior in the Human Female* that in a study of eight thousand women the average frequency for marital coitus by forty years of age was 1.5 times per week and only five percent in this age group made love more than three times a week. In January of 1983

Ladies Home Journal released a survey of eighty-three thousand women whose average age is thirty-five years. This survey revealed that forty-seven percent of these wives have sexual intercourse more than three to five times a week and twenty-seven percent of these wish they could make love more often.

Yankee Doodle keep it up! Yankee Doodle's dandy!

5

NIPPING IN THE BUD

Now consider male semen. (Yes, we must now differentiate between the sexes when discussing semen, because several researchers in female sexuality now believe that during deep orgasms, some females emit a fluid similar to male semen—minus sperm, of course.)

Male semen has a slew of euphemisms used on and off for many centuries. Many of these relate to exotic delicacies, such as: delicious jam, bull gravy, cream, white honey, pudding, baby juice, melted butter, gravy, hot milk, duck-butter, oyster stew, love-liquor, spermatic juice, hot punch, and slime.

Some Eastern cultures believe males should save

their "vital juices" for a special occasion, like two or three emissions for every ten sessions of lovemaking. In contrast, most Western cultures believe if male semen is not emitted there is *no* occasion.

Ancient Eastern sex manuals claimed from the start that females emitted fluid during sexual intercourse. Their fluid was considered inexhaustible and its purpose was to strengthen the male physique. During orgasm a female's fluid (*yin* essence) was thought to be especially rich and, therefore, twice as beneficial for the male's physical well-being. Besides contributing to his general good health, the *yin* essence was a source of rejuvenation and preservation of a male's exhaustible seminal fluid.

The secret of saving vital male juices was, quite literally, a secret. In ancient time, many cults and gurus revealed their methods of retention only to devout followers.

In the ancient East the fountain of youth—for a male—was bubbling over in the vagina of a lusty female, but *only if* he refrained from bubbling along with her.

Usually, Eastern methods for a successful *coitus reservatus* were the use of simple physical distractions, such as stabilizing the breath, opening the eyes wide, closing the mouth and pushing the tongue against the back of the upper teeth, flapping the hands up and down, or, more realistically, gnashing the teeth.

Other solutions were more stirring. A male could, for instance, flip into a backbend or a headstand *if* his penis continued to sip the female's vital juice. Another athletic solution required a male to rhythmically press against the tiny area between his anus and his scrotum with the ball of his left heel between penile gulps. The most difficult method was a form of vampirism. A male was required to retrieve any semen he expended by the dilation, at will, of his urinary bladder—thereby allowing him to draw back into his body the lost fluid. Unfortunately this practice, called *vajroli*, could lead to serious infections of the bladder, so suckers beware.

Today in the West, some males attempt the retention of their semen to prolong sexual pleasure via the "squeeze play" technique. This method was originally created by sex therapists Masters and Johnson to cure premature ejaculation. Masters and Johnson advised the anxious male to practice recognizing his physical reactions just prior to ejaculation. After recognizing these reactions, he was to signal his sex partner, who was in the dominant position, to withdraw his penis and pinch it just below the tip until he had only a partial erection. The anxious male was to continue this pattern until he desired his ejaculation. Men who have tried this technique for *coitus reservertus* claim it works with only one drawback—"it adds a mechanical flavor to lovemaking."

Other than the Masters and Johnson technique, all of the above methods come from Taoist and Tantric treatises on sex that date back to ancient China, India, or Tibet.

In the Old and New Testaments, attitudes toward male semen during copulation are somewhat more inconsistent. At times the Bible appears to consider male semen a precious, sacred thing; at others it is a vile taboo.

The Old Testament's fifth-century-B.C. laws for religious ceremonial purity aptly describe Israel's superstitious fear of bodily emissions, especially sexual:

> And if any man's seed of copulation go out from him, then he shall wash all his flesh in water, and be unclean until the even. And every garment, and every skin, whereon is the seed of copulation, shall be washed with water, and be unclean until even. (Leviticus 15: 16–18)

In Genesis 38: 2–10, semen was considered so sacred that when Onan deliberately dropped his seed on the ground, rather than in the vagina of his slain brother's wife as commanded, the Lord slew him.

Then again, in both Isaiah (7: 14) and Matthew (1: 23) there are agreements that only a virgin shall conceive and bear the son of God, making mortal semen too vile for the conception of a messiah.

The founding fathers of Protestantism broke with early Christian and medieval moralism and declared that sexual intercourse was a healthy habit for the married. Western cultures then adopted a medicinal attitude toward semen. The attitude that sex was healthy eventually convinced many a Western male that the storage of semen would do him great physical and mental harm. This concern—to clean out the plumbing—is prevalent to this day.

But a contrary attitude developed beginning in the Enlightenment, when many a scientist did what he could to stem the flow. Many a medical man preached that every emission was a nail in a male's coffin. As late as Victorian times, the English physician William Acton worried so about the loss of vital energy through sexual activity that *Sexual Variance* tells us:

> He taught that the emission of semen imposed such a great drain on the nervous system that the only way the male could avoid damage was to engage in sex infrequently and then without prolonging the sex act. Males were able to do this because God had created females indifferent to sex to prevent the male's vital energy from being overexpended. Only out of fear that their husbands would desert them for courtesans or prostitutes did most women waive their own natural inclinations and submit to their husband's ardent embraces.

In the last few decades, the scientific attitude has come full circle, with many scientists in various fields assisting in the advancement of the sexual revolution. One example would be a report on a questionnaire sent to over four hundred psychiatrists released in July 1980 by the *Medical Aspects of Human Sexuality*. The questionnaire requested the respondent's personal opinions in several areas of sexuality. One tabulation revealed that thirty-nine percent of the male psychiatrists preferred the coital position of the male on top for the enhancement of their orgasm, forty-seven percent thought the position made no difference, and only six percent preferred the woman above. Female psychiatrists responded to the same question as follows: thirty-eight percent preferred the woman above, thirty-eight percent said the position made no difference, and eighteen percent preferred the male above. To the question, "Are orgasms more intense when lovemaking is brief or prolonged?" replies for prolonged were fifty-two percent of the males against seventy-six percent for females. One other question revealed a large variable between the sexes. Replies to "Are orgasms more pleasurable in youth or when older?" revealed thirty-three percent of the males favoring youth with only nine percent of the females in agreement. Fifty-one percent of the female psychiatrists preferred older (past age thirty-five) against twenty-two percent for the males.

Another scientific assist was Masters and Johnson's 1960 data that disclosed three degrees of erection for the penis. They discovered that during the first, or excitement phase, the hardness of the penile erection varies. They also determined that the longer a male is capable of prolonging the excitement phase and maintaining an intense erection the more skilled a lover he was capable of being.

They termed the second stage the plateau phase. At this point the male organ is fully erect, very warm, with the end of the penis usually developing a reddish purple color. During this phase the Cowper's glands emit just a few drops of semen-containing mucous, but enough to impregnate a female.

The third stage is the orgasmic phase. In this phase the

male has no control over emission. As semen spurts out, the male's heart rate can increase to up to 180 beats per minute, his systolic blood pressure can jump to 100mm of mercury, and his breathing can increase by up to 40 breaths per minute. The muscles at the base of his penis start contracting at 0.8 second intervals with an intensity capable of squirting semen up to two feet in distance.

Now that's a lot of chugging away just to release not quite a teaspoonful of fluid (even if it does contain thirty-two different chemicals, including vitamin C, vitamin B12, fructose, sulfur, zinc, copper, magnesium, potassium, calcium, and other healthy things).

But the best is saved for last. Spermatozoa, the source of life, are emitted from the penis during orgasm along with all of the above goodies. However, despite their powerful potential, spermatozoa comprise only two percent of the total volume of the ejaculate.

Yet what a two percent *if* the male is fairly young and healthy. That's when the sperm count is really loaded. Take this loaded statistic: In males between the ages of twenty and forty-five the sperm count will normally range between 90 and 110 million cells per cubic centimeter. After three days of continence males in this age range average an ejaculation of approximately 3.50cc. From these weighty figures it's easy to compute that sperm are mighty minute— only ⅟₅₀₀th of an inch long.

Sperm resemble no other cell in the human body. They are structured with a definable (under a microscope) head, neck, torso, and tail. In fact so "personable" are they, that biologists in the eighteenth century believed they could see in these tiny cells teeny individual males and females swimming around in a sea of semen, and these biologists theorized that babies were just sperm cells that had increased greatly in size. Biologists named these cells the *homunculi*— the little people.

Not until 1854 was it discovered that it took one male sperm *and* an egg from a female's ovaries to unite with to conceive a child. From prehistoric times until little over a century ago, it was believed that the creation of a human was the magical explosion of the male semen PERIOD. Except in some backward cultures where the role of coitus in reproduction wasn't even discovered.

Scientists have since discovered that mature sperm can develop in boys as early as four years of age, but the average age for American males is between twelve and fourteen years. The youngest reported father was seven years old. There are recorded cases of boys as young as four and five who masturbate with ejaculation and have "wet dreams." In fact, infant males of five and six months have been observed having dry orgasms, and erections are known to occur while a male is still in the uterus.

6

"YOU USED TO COME AT FOUR O'CLOCK, AND NOW YOU COME AT NOON!"

In our expanding cultures the secret of erection on demand has been a search for the fountain of Phallic Youth, from early antiquity till now. And during this vast expanse of time, flappable males have tried a bizarre array of techniques in a search for a solid solution.

The Encyclopedia of Sexual Behavior gives this list (far from current, if we consider the omission of male hormone therapy, or, more recently, penile implant surgery):

. . . baths, salves, smells, parts of animals, blood (especially menstrual blood), powders, pills, creams, oils, narcotics (opium, hashish, marijuana, etc.), ether, electrotherapy, tattooing, erotic pictures, pornographic literature, "dirty" records (not only that reproduce the sounds, vocal and mechanical, such as the rattling noise of bedsprings and even sometimes scatological details), music, mechanical contraptions (fornicating machines, self-satisfiers, pressure pumps for the male organ), *"dames de voyages"* (rubber women), "phallic foods" (foods fashioned in the form of the male and female organs), *"cabinets particuliers"* [the *Encyclopedia* assumes we know this is French for the private dining salon], erotic cookbooks, household articles in sexual forms (lamps, drinking cups, etc.), amulets, charms, and so forth.

Those in dire need of augmentation should research *The Dictionary of Aphrodisiacs* by Harry E. Wedeck, who itemizes and defines in 254 pages erotic stimulants and depressants for the penis. And even this buoyant list, published in 1961, does not include the most visible "upper" of all— the "dirty movie."

Nor does either list include medical science's current solution for problems relating to impotency—the sex therapist, a professional who has discovered and prescribes no more, and probably less, than sex manuals written in ancient times. Considering this turnabout, one could perhaps predict with some surety that the future scientific solution for impotency will be a return to the quaint medical therapies offered centuries back.

For one-upmanship let's take our spade to a few.

In ancient Babylonia, eighth century B.C., a cure for impotency was a combined effort between a physician/priest and the patient. The physician beheaded a male partridge, ate its heart, then combined its blood with water for the patient to drink. Supposedly, the downcast was soon up and tight. Today this treatment would be inconceivable, since the partridge might be on the endangered-species list in a week.

Then there is mandrake, which is mentioned a few times in the Bible indicating its use as an erotic plant. The first mention is Genesis (30: 14–17), where Jacob's barren wife tells him she has hired him with mandrake. With the assist of God and this two-pronged root—that, architecturally, makes the sign of the crotch—Leah is successfully impregnated. Could be mandrake is potent stuff, since Isaac Asimov, in Asimov's *Guide to the Bible*, tabulated that Jacob produced, in total, twelve sons and one daughter (of which two thirds were conceived after Jacob munched on mandrake).

The second reference appears in the Old Testament's sexy Song of Solomon (7: 12–13) when an unknown lover says to her beloved:

> Let us get up early to the vineyards . . . there will I give thee my loves. The mandrakes give a smell, and at our gates [genitals] are all manner of pleasant forms new and old, which I have laid up for thee, O my beloved.

The mandrake, which belongs to the potato family, is indigenous to the Mediterranean area, particularly Palestine. Its ancient Hebrew name is *dudaim*—"dud" meaning love.

The origin of the word *aphrodisiac* aptly comes from the one culture that must have been, from sheer necessity, the primal authority on "uppers." In ancient Greece, every spring prostitutes and courtesans gathered at the city of Corinth to honor, via sexual activities, the love goddess Aphrodite. The festival season, called Aphrodisia, went over with a bang and had many a male attempting to hold up his own with a multitude of sex-crazed women. Street hawkers were soon sold out of fast-food phallic potions and amulets. The best-sellers were those made from the mandrake root.

Mandrake has a persistent history. In medieval time the

plant, in addition to its human form, took up the wail of a banshee. For it was believed that when its roots were taken out of the soil, the mandrake let out an eerie shriek. All who heard its unearthly cry were destined to be killed or go mad—after achieving an erection, of course. It was advised therefore that the plant be uprooted by moonlight with a ritual of prayer *and* the aid of a black dog tied to the foliage, who would tug it from the ground.

If the prospect of plucking a mandrake seems dangerous, a superstitious impotent male might prefer a species of orchid easily identifiable—once uprooted. This exotic erotic plant, so Pliny tells us in writings on the medicinal powers of certain plants, has a double root "shaped like human testicles, which swells and subsides in alternate years." Pliny believed all orchids were a species of satyrion—the plant named after satyrs, who, in human form, represent the Roman god of lust with the mind of a beast.

The power of the satyr plant was so infamous during the time of Nero that the author of the first Western novel, Petronius, titled his libidinous portrait of the decadent society that swayed all of Rome during the first century *The Satyricon*, after this erotic, stimulating plant.

The Satyricon was of course a best-seller for Petronius and still in print to this day. And its hype naturally enhanced the satyr's root's reputation as a cure-all for Roman males when their dart of love went into a dive. Petronius, an audacious rake and satirist, left one more legacy to the history of erotica—his last will and testament gave a detailed report of the multitude of sexual perversions practiced by his patron and friend, Emperor Nero.

Further spade work picks up another erotic stimulant prescribed by Roman physicians during this era. It was touted as a highly effective stimulant; it also smacks of sadomasochism. An impotent male was first advised to eat special erotic foods, such as the fashionable onion, and then pray for assistance from the gods (a request he would soon appreciate). After this ritual the patient was ordered to smear a phallus (dildo) with oil, pepper, and—the real stinger—nettleseed, and then stick it up his anus. While clasping this smarting phallus within, the patient was told to thrash his lower torso with a scourge of nettles (a plant covered with stinging hairs that cause itchy, prickly eruptions on the skin for hours, sometimes days).

And you thought the mandrake let out a shriek!

Scratching the surface we happily unearth another root that because of its appearance became known as a powerful erotic "upper." The ginseng root, a favorite erotic food in ancient China, was an open-sesame device for centuries because it resembled "a man's thighs separated." A similar root was chosen by Indian tribes in Canada for use in erotic potions and worn as jewelry for its mystical, uplifting qualities. What causes two or more unrelated cultures to use almost identical methods to cure man's ailments? Psychologically, theories abound regarding the origin of such behavior, but historically the medical profession defines it as "the doctrine of signatures." Simply put, this means that the more closely a substance in nature resembles a symptom or the affected body part of an ill man, the more likely it is to provide a remedy for what ails him, e.g., the Greek use of orchis, a family of plants whose double bulbs resemble testicles, as a cure for impotency and infertility.

An authority on orchids, Alec Bristow, informs us in *The Sex Life of Plants* that the orchid was "held to have special potent properties to stimulate sexual desires, improve performance and revive flagging powers." The orchid gained this reputation from a primitive conception of its method for reproduction, an unsolved mystery until the early part of this century.

Early naturalists theorized orchids were conceived from the semen of bulls, or other animals, which had dribbled to the ground during mating. This belief was based on the orchid's roots having a striking resemblance to animal and human testes and probably dates back to ancient Greece since the word *orchis* is Greek and translates into Latin as *testis*.

But the true reproductive process of the orchid is far more creative than the imaginings of the early naturalists. Take one species—the bee orchid. This species is unable to form a sexual union with the plant's female organ when its penile "column" is erect—a weird and sorry state for most of the plant's mature life. Only with the sagging of age is the penis united with the plant's vagina. And since Mother Nature frowns upon the vagaries of reproduction in the old age, another method for doing it had to be found if the orchid were to survive with the fittest. The orchid took a step of creative genius: it disguised its bloom as a female bee. What is even more miraculous is the bloom's perfect timing, for it attracted at the height of its sexuality the virginal, inexperienced male bee, days before the hatching season for the female bee.

The orchid's deviant bloom mimicked not only the female bee's markings and color, but the seductive texture of the bee's genitals. So there you have it—a male bee flying around, impatiently awaiting the invasion of B Day, when suddenly he is flagged down by a bigger-than-life "ladylike," vampish, waving bee. He brakes in midair, nosedives down to check out the scent, then zooms in ready for his action. He mounts the blooming "bee," gets his erection, and jigs around searching for the glory hole. What a shock when the virginal male bee discovers, after a thorough probe, that his seductive flirt is minus a bee vagina! In a shocking state he speeds away in search of a vaginal solution for his quandary, unaware that he is the carrier of a sticky yellow mass of pollen. He is again attracted by a gay deceiver and repeats his routine in mounting frustration as the bloom's stigma strips him of his shiny packet. So the virginal male bee becomes, unknowingly, a surrogate penis for one of nature's miracles—cross-fertilization.

A continuing mystery is: how does nature make the orchid so much smarter than the male bee, or many other plants that adopt similar mimicry to sexually attract insects and birds for reproduction and survival as a species?

One plant is a downer in all respects as a penis, and has a scent repellent to humans. As a means of survival this plant has the balls to mimic the human penis in the bloom of a full erection. Tragic to say, this hardy vision of male sexuality, bursting skyward for all to see, stinks to high heaven. It attracts only flies and is appropriately labeled the stinkhorn or the phallic fungi. Its deadly scent—the odor of decaying flesh—attracts carrion flies to the reproductive slime emitting from the head of the phallus. The flies feast on the slime, which is loaded with spores of the stinkhorn. Thus the eggs of the future phallic plants are entrusted to a "womb" of insect excrement. Mother Nature has, at times, a foul sense of humor.

But then so did the physicians in ancient Greece and Rome who prescribed the ingestion of human semen or chopped-up testicles as an erotic potion. Since the gulping of personal semen was an impossibility for an impotent male, physicians prescribed the semen of animals. Also, because human testicles are hard to come by, victims of impotency were advised to place an order with a reliable butcher.

Before taking leave of pseudocannibalism prescribed for males as an erotic stimulant, let's examine one that makes old wives pale—the vampiring of vaginas of virgins. Since ancient times, elderly studs have been medically advised to sample the vaginal fluids of virgins in their original containers whenever there is a noticeable slackening in their erections. Of course, like many medical mysteries, this cure for impotency has its ups and downs. Take this royal flop from the Bible (I Kings 1: 1–4):

Now King David was old and stricken in years; and
they covered him with clothes, but he gat no heat.
Wherefore his servants said unto him, Let there be
sought for my lord the king a young virgin: and let her
stand before the king, and let her cherish him, and let
her lie in thy bosom, and that my lord the king may get
heat. So they sought for a fair damsel throughout all the
coast of Israel . . . and brought her to the king. And the
damsel was very fair, and cherished the king, and min-
istered to him: but the king knew her not.

Let's move on to this savory combination: a comeup-
pance debate on the comparative merits of eggs or onions as
a long-lasting aphrodisiac. *The Perfumed Garden* gives this
comparison report:

The member of Abou el Heiloukh has remained erect
For thirty days without a break, because he did eat onions.
Abou el Heidja has deflowered in one night
Once eighty virgins, and he did not eat or drink between . . .
Mimoun, the negro, never ceased to spend his sperm, while he
For fifty days without a truce the game was working.
How proud he was to finish such a task!
For ten days more he worked it, not yet was he surfeited,
But all this time he ate but yolk of egg and bread.

Before we dig up drugs and external forms of sexual
stimulation, the aficionado of aphrodisiacs might be interested to learn which, of all the plants, 'tis said can raise the
dead. It has been rumored that if the mandrake root grows
beneath the gallows, a hanged man's penis will rise again
while he hangs loose in the noose. And not only does the root
bestow the last "upper," it also gives one final shot at
ejaculation. Naturally, most physicians puncture this balloon, claiming the true cause of a hanged male's erection
and ejaculation is the surge of blood raging into the genital
area after the trauma of a violent respiratory attack. Yet
Havelock Ellis came up with an entirely different explana-

tion. Ellis says there are many recorded cases of sexual stimulation as a result of suspension and strangulation, which "has always been a conspicuous part of the whole process of tumescence [swelling] and detumescence, of the struggles of courtship and of its climax . . . and that any restraint upon respiration . . . tends to heighten the state of sexual excitement . . ." Ellis goes on to quote a source saying "people suffering from lung disease are often erotically inclined."

Of course death on the gallows or the contraction of a lung disease to achieve an upper could only be the choice for a raging masochist.

In a hierarchy of handy maneuvers to up the penis, at the top of the peak perches masturbation, sometimes in duet but more often solo. A smacking second is fellatio. Third is the broad sphere of voyeurism, which spies from many views (e.g., "dirty" movies, books, and magazines; burlesque shows; "peeping"; etc.) on the nudity or the sexual activities of others.

Topping this degenerate mass is masochism, which makes tracks all over the place. There are several primitive manifestations attesting to the ecstasy experienced from physical pain. First there is the human's association of animalism with the sexual acts often illustrated physically by the writhing in pain many animals exhibit during mating. Another is forbidden excitement, especially when there are threats of severe punishment—a story as old as Eden. Finally, there are the masochistic actions taken, and recommended for others, by religious zealots to achieve transcendental heights of awareness.

Pain has a lot going for it, something recognized as far back as ancient Greece by those who organized the orgiastic festivals for Aphrodite. To stir the senses and create the atmosphere for a sexual orgy, the courtesan/priestesses would perform erotic whippings on supplicant males before the altars of their temples. It was considered a smash act. In the

Orient, where Aphrodite and her fests were unknown, flagellation was esteemed a breeze for males whose flags were fluttering at half-mast. Also, in isolated tribes around the globe, flogging rituals were employed to inspire virility and increase sexual aggression.

Not till the end of the nineteenth century did medical science discover flagellation was a dread disease. Herr Doctor Krafft-Ebing stopped "clamping down" on masturbators long enough to christen whipping, and other forms of sexual stimulation derived from the sensation of physical pain, *masochism*. Krafft-Ebing chose a fellow Teut to carry the bannerhead of this new disease, Ritter Leopold von Sacher-Masoch, author famed for his books and stories describing the artistry required for such an experience. Herr Doctor considered his christening a put-down of the author's torrid tales: instead, of course, there was an immediate increase in sales.

Soon best-sellers for the Victorian underground presses were books describing the Barnum-and-Bailey-style productions put on in brothels throughout Europe which specialized in flagellation. The settings, costumes, and equipment were opulent and imaginative, creating the effect of a three-ring circus. There were trapezes and swings, blocks and pillories, furs and spangles, corsets and garters, spiky heels and boots, tiaras and satin, rabid nuns and scolding schoolmarms. Brothels dripped with a variety of reinforcement equipment capable of jacking up the penis of the most jaded gent. The madams of these brothels made it impossible not to twitch, for their customers were lashed with everything from spiked cat-o'-nine-tails to leather thongs, from heavy whips to serious chains.

Contemporary psychological studies claim that a high percentage of those males addicted to flagellation are successful in their careers, highly ambitious, and achieve their goals with relative ease. Perhaps those who "sacrifice" and "suffer" to acquire their triumphs find small need for additional pain.

A sadist, understandably, has a painful problem maintaining a permanent relationship sexually, other than with a wailing masochist. He goes in almost constant search of a victim necessary for his erotic arousal. Even the brothel, an old standby for most sexual deviants, rarely seeks his business, and when they take the gamble, their fee is exorbitant.

Many sadists wind up as jailbirds. Indeed, sadism is named after an infamous jailbird, the Marquis de Sade, who was imprisoned for kidnapping a prostitute and forcing her to submit to repeated beatings and other nasties. While in prison during the French Revolution and later confined by the emperor Napoleon to an insane asylum, de Sade wrote novels and plays defining in brutal detail the endless orgies he could personally recommend to those who shared his voracious appetite for the infliction of pain as an erotic stimulant.

In his will, de Sade requested with rare humility that his ashes be scattered so that "the traces of my grave disappear from the face of the earth, as I flatter myself that my memory will be effaced from the minds of men." De Sade's books indeed proved hotter than his ashes, for his coercive tales secured for the Marquis a perpetual memorial—citing him in psychological and medical texts as the definitive authority on the broad aspects for quenching the thirst of vampirical sadism.

To wind up external acts used as aphrodisiacs there are two further oddities (to those unafflicted).

Fetishism was "discovered" as a degenerative disease in 1888 by the French psychologist Alfred Binet. The term stems from the Latin *facere*, to make, to fascinate. *The Encyclopedia of Sex* gives a fascinating list: "shoe-fetishists, glove-fetishists, fur-fetishists, silk-fetishists, velvet-fetishists, lingerie-fetishists, leather-fetishists, or hair-fetishists."

Fetishism is almost exclusively a male aberration; there are no two ways about it, according to most studies.

A predominant psychoanalytical theory claims that fetishism is a basic male sexual deviance suffered by males who refuse to acknowledge that females do not have penises. Analysts' reasoning goes like this: Certain small boys become traumatized upon their discovery that there are penisless creatures. Hiding their terror and disgust, these boys conclude that all females are, in some mysterious way, castrated. Penalized with fright, these tiny ones go in constant fear of some unknown penis snatcher. To ease these fears, they fantasize about objects that could possibly be attached to the castrated victims as a subsitute for their lost genitals. The objects chosen by small boys are close at hand, have a sensuous texture, and are usually phallic in shape or color. As the boys enter adolescence and early manhood, their childish secret terror becomes sublimated, with the fantasized phallus emerging as the superior erotic object. In short they refuse to acknowledge the existence of the vagina.

Most psychologists and many psychiatrists consider this theory a nonsensical nightmare—one only an analyst could dream up. They claim instead the basic cause of fetishism stems from an infant or small child becoming deeply attached to an object, rather than a person, that incites his initial sexual arousal. Thus when sexual gratification from this object continues over a long period of time, the child begins to associate the erotic stimulus with his sexual goal. And, since males psychologically receive more erotic stimulation from tactile experiences than do females, fetishism is predominantly a male sexual deviance. The lengthy process for achieving this erotic stimulation is called "imprinting."

Imprinting was first discovered in certain species of birds. Since then zookeepers have recognized it as a serious mating problem in several species of animals (i.e., the panda and the gorilla). In captivity certain animals are isolated from the opposite sex as a precautionary measure. This segregation during the early years causes these animals, in the mating season, to seek sexual gratification from those who nourish and care for them (experimentation in imprinting also proves an animal can be trained to relate sexually to an object). Author Desmond Morris, among other zoologists, tells us that during captivity these animals eventually begin to consider themselves people rather than members of their own species. A recent example of this is the toe-tapping, arm-flapping love affair between a male West Coast ornithologist and a female Wisconsin whooping crane.

The whooping crane is high on the endangered-species list for many reasons, only one of which is an adamant refusal to mate in captivity. Another reason is that in the wild, cranes mate for life and then do it only after cautious scrutiny and much ritual. These instincts apparently are carried by the crane into captivity, as the following bird's-eye view of romance will demonstrate.

Tex, the female crane, was raised from a chick in a zoo and had developed a snapping dislike of the males of her species, especially during the mating season. At the age of eight, in 1975, Tex fell head over wings in love with the visiting director of the International Crane Foundation, ornithologist George Archibald. Tex, known for her savvy, chose to whoop it up only with a mover and a shaker.

George, after periodic visits, quickly ascertained he was the chosen one when Tex began attacking anyone who interrupted their chats and pats. With the approach of the spring mating season George, in a unique experiment, determined to take advantage of Tex's erotic fixation for him. After Tex was artificially inseminated with crane semen, George moved into her enclosure. His goal was to get Tex aroused sexually so that she would produce an egg. In the mating of cranes this is accomplished only through the energetic ritual of dance. For days during three mating seasons, 1977 through 1979, George flapped his arms, tapped his toes, and leaped high into the air, his "beak" aimed to the heavens. Doing the same, Tex jived right along, having a ball—without dropping an egg.

Finally, in 1982, George determined to give his all. He moved into Tex's enclosure for the seven-week annual spring mating season. Tex was in heaven. They danced every day, sometimes several times a day. Until one day Tex released her egg. True blue George remained after the egg was removed for safekeeping. He assisted Tex, as would the mate of her species, in building a nest and took his turn sitting, perched on a camp stool, for three weeks hatching the spurious egg.

The chick from the bona fide egg, hatched by surrogate hen, was christened Gee Whiz: Gee in honor of Dr. Gee who provided the crane semen from a wildlife center in Texas and Whiz for that toe-tapper erotic George Archibald, the chosen one who followed through.

But George did not return to Wisconsin in the spring of 1983 to flap and tap. Tex had been killed the previous winter. She was found one morning in her enclosure, mauled and partially eaten by some unknown four-legged critter, who, we hope, died an agonizing death after attempting to digest such an exotic dish.

The other supposed deviancy used for penile stimulation is transvestism, cross-dressing, a phenomenon separate from transsexuality, described later in this book. Some therapists claim transvestism is closely aligned with fetishism, possibly a spin-off. Again, transvestism is almost solely practiced by males, and theories of its origins are similar to those of fetishism—early sexual conditioning or fear of castration. Supposedly, the possibility of castration is a horror for transvestites since the source of their sexual pleasure is their male genitals. Cross-dressing for a transvestite is an erotic stimulant, a fantasy unaccompanied by a desire for a vagina.

Finally, in the past decade, due to modern technology, an easing of regulations for advertising in magazines and newspapers, and an increasing tendency for personal noninvolvement, yet another aphrodisiac has come to our ears—telephone erotica. While some aggressive studs snicker, others hail this erotic device for its remote control, simplicity, safety, inexpensiveness (in comparison to hourly rates in a brothel or costly illegal drugs), legality, and availability—within seconds throughout the United States, necessitating only a major credit card and a telephone. For a minimal cost, $20 or $30, plus an additional charge if long distance, a caller receives a thirty-minute monologue of sexual obscenities slanted toward his favorite fantasy. The majority of callers are males with a preference for female tale-bearing.

In the 1920s ear sex was labeled by the psychiatric community as a sexual deviance, *coprolalia*, a fixation with the use of obscenities—the love of filth.

Previous to phone sex, lovers of filth had a problem, since a siren's wail of obscenities, besides being difficult to transmit, took a combination of skills (vocal cords of velvet crusted with lust, a racy imagination, an unbiased spirit, and a glowing respect for melodrama) which rarely paid off. Today phone sex is big bucks. Take one for instance. In February of 1983 Ma Bell connected with an additional $150,000 *per week* when a girlie magazine in New York City used a fifty-seven-second sexy earful as a promotional gimmick.

Today the only frustration a coprolaliac comes within earshot of is a busy signal.

Along with gnawing roots and dallying with deviance since preantiquity, males have teetered on the seesaw of unstable drug ingestion for a penile "upper." Toying with drugs, on a rare occasion, has steadied some shaky timbers, yet, used on a regular basis, these same drugs topple the sturdiest totems. Tragically, there is a long list of lethal drugs males, in search of a cocksure stimulant, will experiment with.

Inventors of the first written language, the ancient Sumerians, already knew the flagrant poppy that produces opium (and heroin and morphine and codeine) as "the plant of joy." Opium, unknown in the Far East until the seventh century, was first introduced to China as a medicinal narcotic. With increased use over centuries the poppy seed's reputation for inducing sensual exhilaration bloomed. But poppy rot didn't set in until a new fad swept China—pipe smoking, the new fashion in Europe after Columbus brought its tawny weed from the New World, was soon wafted into China by Portuguese traders during the seventeenth century. As the importation of tobacco halfway around the world was prohibitive and time consuming, the Chinese improvised by smoking the potent poppy. Since opium smoking reduced inhibitions, increased erotic dreaming, and occasionally provided an impotent male with an uplifting experience, it was soon touted as the ultimate aphrodisiac. Unfortunately, those accompanying erotic daydreams soon became more entrancing than the reality of sexual intercourse. In little more than a century, a devastating percentage of China's vast population, both male and female, was smoldering in a dreamland of sexual extinction: in 1729 China imported two hundred chests of the powdered drug annually; in another century the total had flamed to over sixty thousand chests. An alarmed government, fearful its population was going up in smoke, banned further imports. The British, the largest exporters to China, snarled that the government's ruling would destroy the balance of trade in the Orient—which it did—and, before you could spit in the ocean, a war was on, followed by Opium War II. Not until the early twentieth century did China awake from its three-century nightmare and win its internal war against the deadly dream of the poppy.

Today its nodding blossom still stinks in many areas of the world. Poppy fields blaze their buds in remote regions of Laos, Thailand, Burma, Pakistan, Iran, Turkey, and Mexico. Currently the big push is on for a powerful opium derivative, the deadly "downer" heroin.

In our own country the fashionable "upper" in the past few years is the illegal drug cocaine, an extract of the coca plant, blatantly exported out of several South American countries. Coke is expensive; you pay through the nose. Yet, while the drug wholesales at $50,000 a kilo (the size of a small pizza) sales continue to boom in our high-living, sexually brainwashed, energy-conscious U.S.A.

For sexually wavering studs who want to be up to snuff, a sniff of coke is touted as the ultimate erotic stimulant. In addition pushers hype a stirring combo: after a snort, a stud's towering turn-on will be gyrated into spiraling orgasms sparked from his sex partner's blasting reaction to the insertion of his coke-daubed penis.

So what could be bad? For the penis plenty. Coke as a penile "upper" is a snow job. The director of the Haight Ashbury Free Medical Clinic in San Francisco, Dr. David E. Smith, found "heavy users generally have erectile failure or experience total loss of sexual desire." Other therapists discovered that habitual users of cocaine were addicted psychologically to the drug since withdrawal caused deep depression often accompanied by suicidal tendencies.

In addition to the above, "downers" are another possible devastator—leading to permanent sexual apathy. This author interviewed a thirty-one-year-old male cocaine addict in May of 1983. The still young male had a history of coke addiction for over four years that had accelerated from snorting to free-basing it. Now "clean" of coke and a bankroll (for the last two years he paid $500 a day to get high) he fears he has become a psychological celibate. Since his withdrawal from cocaine some three years ago he says he has "absolutely no interest in sex at all despite being physically potent." When asked what he attributed this to he replied, "No orgasm can compete with the euphoric state one gets while free-basing cocaine. I am burned out erotically. Permanently."

Neither psychologically or physically addictive (due to its poisonous nature), but an undisputed penile upper speared with convulsive pain is the lethal powder made from dried beetles found in most of southern Europe. The beetle drug, known to ancient physicians as the blasting diuretic cantharis, was quixotically tagged "Spanish fly" by Yanks in the late nineteenth century. Because the potent drug caused an immediate erection through inflammation of the genitals, unscrupulous physicians promoted it as a dynamite cure for impotency. And, before you could wave your stalk, the hydraulic drug was being black-marketed as an erotic potion. Its good point—that the beetle drug aimed the penis in the right direction—was upheld; the problem was that the erection was an agonizing, irreversible, explosive event that often resulted in insanity and death. Which resulted in a collapse in sales. Pushers quickly switched their hype to claim the beetle drug was still a pick-up for studs since it was capable of turning any female, regardless of age, into a nymphomaniac.

By the eighteenth century, *The Dictionary of Aphrodisiacs* tells us, cantharis was "widely used as a sexual stimulant. Cooked in bisquits, cakes and pastry, and inserted in candies and chocolates." Proof of sexual poisoning lies, again, with the sadistic de Sade, who fed bonbons laced with the beetle drug to prostitutes. They petered out permanently after one of his tailspinning orgies.

Are the lethal effects of the beetle drug, regardless of

sex, an old wives' tale enhanced by paranoid puritans? Not likely. This author recently interviewed a partygoer who, a few years earlier, witnessed the agonizing, convulsive deaths of two fellow guests after a punch bowl was underhandedly spiked with Spanish fly (a party pooper carryover from the drug-haranguing sixties—lacing of punch bowls with LSD, still another hallucinogen used as an erotic stimulant).

Seldom do the hazy pipe dreams of users—or pushers—of drugs, legal or illicit, concur with scientific findings. This is especially true when drugs are analyzed as erotic stimulants. A recent example is a report on the effectiveness of several illicit drugs that had gained reputations as aphrodisiacs during the seventies. A professor of health care sciences and medicine at George Washington University, Thomas E. Plemme, MD, weeded out the following dope, from several studies, on penile uppers:

> Marijuana: has little influence on the sex act and no evidence that it increased sex drive or frequency of intercourse.
> Heroin: that narcotic use increases impotence in most dependent users. Also, males who use narcotics frequently note delay or failure of ejaculation and a patient sometimes uses the drug for this purpose.
> Barbiturates: behave precisely as alcohol does—inhibitions are lowered, euphoria ensues, ejaculations may be delayed, and impotence can result if large quantities are used.
> Cocaine: regular use almost certainly deters the sex act, often resulting in impotence. There were, also, spontaneous erections and priapism [a continued painful erection].
> Psychedelics: occasionally patients become involved in erotic hallucinations, but they are not acted out. Patients report that taking LSD to initiate sexual relations is useless because the user can't remain focused on what he started to do.

Amphetamine: the one drug that is clearly documented as showing increased frequency and scope of sexual activity. Still, during a "high" the male user is often incapable of an erection. Only during a "crash" is interest in sex enhanced.

Penile implants are the most recent technological solution for certain forms of impotency, but for an immediate solution, the owner of an aging, pooped penis might consider the latest word from sex therapists—"Use it or lose it." The data on which they base this latest therapy originates from studies on the frequency of sexual intercourse in the lives of senior citizens. Male seniors claim the more sex they have, the more often they are capable of it.

But other studies by sex researchers claim boredom with one's partner accounts for most of male impotency. Still others claim too much sex can lead to a burn-out, especially when there is a swift and constant change in sexual partners.

After all these ups and downs, some might find the following report on abstinence, continence, chastity, and celibacy a sensible rest for the wicked—or a cover-up solution for the impotent.

7

THRUST NOT OR FOREVER HOLD YOUR PIECE

Those in search of moist inlets will find sexual abstinence a dry issue. Nevertheless, it's been around as long as humans and sex—almost. And, since it is a virtue in many religions and an ideal in some philosophies, it was traditionally considered an honorable put-down for human penises.

However, things have now changed; the 1982 *Encyclopaedia Britannica* cites sexual abstinence (along with rape, incest, necrophilia, and homosexuality) under Sexual Deviations, while celibacy and chastity are categorized separately as "legitimate" topics.

The *Britannica* defines abstinence as the conscious

avoidance of sexual relations by means of masturbation, fantasy, disguised sexual excitement (religious frenzies), or total self-denial. Its various motivations are: "extreme commitment to a moral or intellectual purpose . . . fear of punishment from one's conscience . . . [or] rare persons who, though biologically normal, are effortlessly abstinent." And, as "a test of motivation and respectable offering to higher powers . . . pursued for thousands of years in almost every culture. Its value in focusing energy into other productive channels . . . is as strong today as in earlier eras." *Britannica* also adds: "Although masturbation itself *may not be sexually deviant in a statistical sense, the fantasies accompanying it usually are.*" (Emphasis added.)

Celibacy is defined as the state of being unmarried as a result of a sacred vow. And: "Celibacy has existed in some form or another throughout all man's religious history and in virtually all major religions of the world."

Chastity is defined as the "abstention from unlawful sexual intercourse, or total abstention from sexual intercourse . . . most commonly for religious motives."

Britannica skips continence, but it is defined in the Funk & Wagnalls (1946) *New Standard Dictionary* as: "Self-restraint with respect to desires, appetites, and passions; especially, self-restraint with respect to the sexual passion, either in celibacy or in marriage."

Who invented sexual abstinence? And whyever did they? Historians tell us the origin of sexual abstinence is superstition, beginning with prehistoric man's search for methods to appease the mysterious forces of nature. Bewildered, often frightened, primitive man invented activities to ward off bad luck or to gain a particular objective. Thus, in a life with few pleasures or possessions, the sacrifical action became a means to barter and exchange with unseen powers, and withdrawal from sexual intercourse often topped the list, since primitive man had little else to offer.

With the passage of centuries, these superstitions were accepted into religious activities. And it goes full circle, for some religious rituals have become everyday superstitious acts, among them keeping your fingers crossed, an early Christian act for making the sign of the cross.

Vedism, primeval Hinduism and possibly the world's earliest formalized religion, conceived the first religious ascetic—the celibate guru. During the fourth century B.C., the founder of Buddhism, Gautama (Buddha is a title—"the enlightened one"—not a proper name), abandoned a sheltered life as a wealthy Indian prince, his wife, and a newborn son, after realizing all living things were destined for illness and death. At the time, he was an unenlightened twenty-nine years of age. Gautama's search for a solution to this dreary fate took six years of wandering and study as a religious ascetic. Then, sitting cross-legged, meditating under a banyan tree, he discovered "the great Enlightenment" (extinction or blowing out). Man's liberation from suffering and death could be achieved through the extinction of personal desire (yep! sexual, too) and individual consciousness.

Buddha's enlightenment became the basis for the Buddhist faith and the origin of celibate communal living or the monastic existence, which continues in many forms in most areas of the world today (though the vow of celibacy predominates, it is not universal).

Still, the road to enlightenment for Buddha possibly had its pleasures, for some historians claim Buddha died from an overdose of psychedelic mushrooms.

Jainism (*Jain* meaning "conqueror") was another ascetic Indian faith which advocated a celibate monastic life as a means of salvation. It also sanctified nudity, for an upper caste of Jainist monk was required to wander naked, offering the hollow of his hand as an alms bowl. A lower caste was allowed to wear a loincloth and to carry an alms bowl, a piece of cloth not to exceed a yard and a half, and a "sweeper" to clear his path so he might not injure even the lowliest insect. Both castes were forbidden to look at a woman, for "they are to monks what a cat is to a chicken."

The most illustrious example of Hindu asceticism—for the Western world—was the twentieth-century Indian leader Mahatma Gandhi, who took the vow of celibacy though continuing to live with his wife.

Historian Stanley J. Pacion tells us that Gandhi

> believed his former life of the passions was a trap, that they controlled him rather than he controlling them. The joy of being his own man, the inner happy sense of liberty, would soon lead Gandhi to create a new image for himself . . . [and] . . . more important . . . were the results of Gandhi's sexual credo on India. Because he was revered as a saint among the people, his unconditional rejection of any form or practice of birth control soon became the dominant belief of the land. To be sure, Gandhi would never license unchecked intercourse. But his insistence that sexual relations be limited to the number three or four during the entire marriage was an unreachable ideal even for the most devoted of his followers.

Many believe Gandhi was a misogynist, for he forbade, unsuccessfully, his sons to marry. One of his four sons, Harilal, embittered with Gandhi's celibate views, was driven to alcoholism and writing hostile publications about his father's political, religious, and marital beliefs. Others cite as evidence that Gandhi was *not* a misogynist his insistence, as an aging man, on being cradled in the laps of naked young—preferably beautiful—virgin women to cure (temporarily) his recurrent attacks of violent trembling.

Sexual asceticism surfaced in the Western world about the middle of the third century B.C. It was kicked off by religious cults in ancient Greece who became disenchanted when their Olympian gods failed to prevent the decay of

Greek political and military dominance and the corresponding rise of the hated, hedonistic Romans. The predominant cult was Orphism, which advocated the abstention from meat, wine, and sexual intercourse. Devotees of Orphism despised all things sensuous and exalted life in the next world.

These ascetic cults never made an impressive dent in the religious mainstream. Their austere views on sexuality and sex were just too drastic a change in lifestyle for the sensuous Greeks, who for centuries had been living a libidinous existence with the approval of their gods.

However, by the end of the third century B.C. theories of sexual abstinence for the liberation of the intellect began to appear in Greek philosophy. Even earlier Socrates had argued that man's highest goal was the freedom of the mind and that the practice of chastity was an essential condition for attaining this freedom. Socrates also theorized that, although he was married (to a shrew) and had three sons, he lived with his wife *only* to teach himself self-control. Shrewdly, he never put any of this in writing.

Through his writings, Socrates's student Plato preserved Socratic ideals. And while there is no doubt of Plato's Socratic beliefs, there is room for speculation that his dedication to their preservation might be traced to a guilty conscience. The day the Athenian government executed Socrates by poison, Plato was "indisposed." Later, dutifully—and beautifully—Plato described this day in his dialogue *Phaedo*, which dramatically details Socrates's slow death while surrounded by other students and friends.

Plato (his true name was Aristocles; Plato was a nickname meaning "broad-shouldered") also founded the Academy, the first think tank. It was there that ascetic beliefs in political, communal, and personal existence were explored and absorbed by students and intellects. As the Academy was the first permanent community for the study and discussion of humane and exact sciences, it is considered the first university. Of course, this school was not coed and there were no panty raids.

In two other dialogues, the *Symposium* and the *Phaedrus*, Plato describes the limitations of desirous love—eros. The *Symposium* claims that love in its crudest form is a passion to achieve immortality through the offspring of a beautiful person, while spiritual forms of love lead to the discovery of the "Form of the Good"—a supreme form standing above all others.

In the *Phaedrus* Plato describes two kinds of love: the sacred (the mind) and the profane (the body). He compares them with two winged steeds, one white, one black (guess which one), under the control of a charioteer (the soul) whose aim is to discipline the unruly black steed so he might run in harmony with the white thoroughbred. After achieving harmony, the chariot would take flight from the earth and mount to the company of the gods.

Will Durant, in *The Life of Greece*, claims that when Plato talks of human love in the *Phaedrus*, he means homosexual love, and that "the disputants in his Symposium agree on one point—that love between man and man is nobler and more spiritual than love between man and woman."

While Greek philosophy reached new heights through the development of Plato's ideals, the general populace sensibly went on with their blanket drills, until four centuries later when the early Christian fathers adopted Plato's ascetic beliefs in an attempt to throttle the pagan world.

The early Christians adopted many rituals and some beliefs from the Judaic faith. But their attitudes toward sexuality and sexual intercourse were from the opposite ends of a pole. The ancient Judaic faith revered the sexual act to the point of law. A prime example is ancient Israel's marriage license and ceremony, which consisted of an agreement for a union between the newlyweds' parents and consummation of the sexual act by the couple, which, in itself, was the marriage ceremony.

And while Judaism had its own religious ascetics, the Nazirites, none of their vows related to sexual abstinence. Instead, these holy men, said to be endowed with special psychic and physical powers, were required to abstain from eating certain foods, drinking wine, cutting their hair, and— the easy one—touching a corpse. Samson, you may have guessed, was a Nazirite and considered a holy warrior until he divulged to the temptress Delilah the secret of his strength and was shorn.

The Talmud concept of a sex calendar is yet another example. It is described in *The Prepared Table* (Shulhan 'arukh) by the sixteenth-century rabbi Joseph Karo in his definitive codification of Talmudic law:

> Each man is obliged to perform his marital duty according to his strength and according to his occupation. Gentlemen of leisure should perform their marriage obligation every night. Laborers who are employed in the city where they reside should perform their duty twice weekly, but if they are employed in another city, once a week. Donkey drivers . . . once a week; camel-drivers, once in thirty days; sailors, once in six months. As for scholars, it is obligatory for them to have intercourse once a week, and it is customary for this to be on Friday nights. (Eben-Ha-Ezer, 76:1)

In the Old Testament there are also many indications (i.e., the Song of Solomon) that sexual intercourse outside of marriage (minus the license of parental consent?) did not break Judiac law.

Yet the Christian New Testament expounds entirely different attitudes. This is well illustrated in the writings of Saint Paul, who apparently considered even marriage one short step above the pits, for he says, " 'Tis better to marry than to burn." And Paul goes even further in 1 Thessalonians (4: 3–5):

> For this is the will of God, *even* your sanctification that ye should abstain from fornication: That every one of you should know how to possess your vessel in sanctification and honour; Not in lust or concupiscence, even as Gentiles which know not God.

Perhaps the explanation for Paul's trashing of sexual intercourse came from his birthplace and hometown, Tarsus, which was the home base for many ascetic Stoic philosophers. For Paul, though trained as a rabbi (but working as a tentmaker), was said to have been proud of his knowledge of Greek culture and philosophy. Still, the populace of Tarsus was not above taking a peek at a sexy piece. For example, a half-century before the birth of Paul, in 41 B.C. Cleopatra sailed into this city's harbor and pulled out all her stops. She was rowed to shore by scantily clad handmaidens as she languished on shiny golden sheets, beneath purple silken sails, dressed (?) as Venus. This class act was put on in an all-out effort to swamp Marc Antony, who immediately sold himself downriver.

After his conversion to Christianity, Paul began his voluminous writings to inform early Christians of the imminence of the Second Coming of the Savior, to be followed by the Last Judgment. Paul claimed that all those who hoped to be saved had to be pure in thought and deed. And, indeed, sexual abstinence got top preference, for the first to be saved would be virgins—either male or female, since heaven was nonsexist, other than its upper echelon, *naturally*. Next on Paul's list of those to be saved were full-time celibates. Last place was reserved for those who had married. Sex without marriage put anyone in hell.

Paul's chaste Platonic theories got wide approval from

the first-century Christians, who were mostly of a lower so-cioeconomic status and who detested the hedonistic upper classes. With the spread of Christian idealism, a collision with the decadent, pagan Roman Empire was inevitable.

Early Christians were determined reformists urging rev-olution, not only in religion, but in lifestyles and politics—such as a refusal to serve in the army, a *big* no-no in the Roman Empire. Not surprising, therefore, Roman leaders began taking extreme measures to destroy the Christians. A vivid example of this persecution is described by the Roman senator and historian Tacitus when he tells us how easily Nero switched his blame for the nine-day burning of Rome on to the Christians and his exquisite cruelty in punishing them:

> Some were covered with the skins of wild beasts, and left to be devoured by dogs; others were nailed to crosses; numbers of them were burned alive; many, cov-ered with inflammable matter, were set on fire to serve as torches during the night.

Nero took great pride in being a creative killer, but as a personal hit man his luck ran out when he took on his mother, Agrippina. After five attempts to rid himself of her interference in the supervision of his empire by killing her, Nero finally hired a servant to do the job. Nero's first three attempts were, for him, uninspired—he used quick-acting poison. His fourth was fanciful but inaccurate; he recon-structed the ceiling in Agrippina's bedroom so that it would fall and crush her to death. But Nero's fifth attempt was far out. He installed a collapsible bottom in her boat. It made a killing with the boat, but when it sank (Will Cuppy in *The Decline and Fall of Practically Everybody* tells us) Agrippina proved she could swim like a mink.

The next big push for sexual abstinence came from the

fourth-century theologians Ambrose, Jerome, Basil, and Augustine, each of these whom had a specific target. The earliest, Ambrose, took on sex in marriage. In fact, he took on marriage itself. For Ambrose advocated austere asceticism and glorified virginity. He borrowed from Stoic philosophy the notion that reason must overtake passion, especially sexual passion. In his sermons Ambrose preached that the best course for a woman was virginity, for as a virgin she could then redeem the sin her parents committed in conceiving her.

Jerome came next. He asserted that sex was dirty. Jerome wrote often of "virgins that were squalid with dirt." And that dirt "both epitomized the sexual act and the therapeutic process by which the virgin concealed her charms." *The Natural History of Love* says that Jerome went even further, decreeing sexual passion within marriage an unholy state and "such was the nature of sexual love—even within marriage—that just after it, neither prayer nor communion was possible." In the seventh century this startling doctrine became Church dogma when a manual for priests, the Penitential, ordered, "Those who are joined together in matrimony should abstain from cohabitation three nights before receiving communion."

Jerome should be crowned the patron saint of pornographers—for the invention that sex is dirty makes them more money than they can shake their sticks at.

Basil was a worrier. He organized the first Christian monasteries and was ever fearful of the distractions of homosexuality. *Sexual Variance* quotes Basil warning the young monk:

> At meals take a seat far away from your young brother;
> in lying down to rest, let not your garments be neighbor
> to his; rather have an elderly brother between you.
> When a young brother converses with you or is opposite

you in choir, make your response with your head bowed
lest perchance by gazing fixedly into his face the seed of
desire be implanted in you by the wicked sower and you
reap sheaves of corruption and ruin.

But the greatest campaigner during the fourth century
for the celibate life was Augustine, a real backer of Original
Sin ("the revolt of the flesh against the spirit"). Before his
conversion to Christianity, Augustine was a member of the
Manichaean church, whose "elect" were celibate monks.
However, Augustine chose, at the time, to be "unelected,"
since he was living with a young concubine and admits his
constant prayer was "Lord, give me chastity and continency,
but do not give them yet."

Later, in his autobiography, Augustine describes his
growing self-contempt after learning of the heroic actions of
ascetic Christians and claims his release from the powers of
sexuality came when a child's voice told him "take up and
read." By chance Augustine chose a book beside him which
fell open to these dreary words of Paul telling the Romans,
"Make no provisions for the flesh, to fulfill the lust . . ." (Romans 13: 14). So imperative an event was this to the guilt-
ridden Augustine that he converted to Christianity that day
and took—finally—the vow of celibacy.

There is no hint that Augustine ever attempted other
forms of abstinence, which, in religious circles, were quite
the rage. For instance, in their monasteries ascetic Syrian
monks attempted to abstain from sleep by—literally—hanging in there, tied by ropes and dangling all through the night
in awkward, dangerous positions. And a collection of anecdotes by desert ascetics describes their preoccupation with
sex and a sure cure-all, probably inspired by the aforementioned words of Paul to the Romans:

. . . a young monk tormented by sexual daydreams asks
a wise old monk: "I entreat thee to explain to me how

thou hast never been harried by lust." The old man replies: "Since the time that I became a monk, I have never given myself my fill of bread, or of water, nor of sleep, and tormenting myself with appetite for these things whereby we are fed, I was not suffered to feel the stings of lust."

And another anecdote describes the wishful thinking of a celibate priest about to give up the ghost:

> . . . who [after taking his orders] . . . parted from his wife, although he loved her. Forty years later, when he lay in a coma, dying of ague, his aged wife visited him and bent over his bed. In great fervor of spirit . . . he burst out, saying: "Get thee away, woman, a little fire is yet left; take away the straw."

Sex, according to Augustine, had damned us all since Original Sin first sprouted in the Garden of Eden.

In his major work, *The City of Hope*, Augustine describes how he believed "innocent" conception would have to occur in Eden:

> In Paradise, then, generative seed would have been sown by the husband, and the wife would have conceived . . . by deliberate and not by uncontrollable lust. After all, it is not only our hands and fingers, feet and toes, made up by joints and bones that we move at will, but we can also control the flexing and stiffening of muscles and nerves. . . . Some people . . . can make their ears move, either one at a time or both together. . . . There are individuals who can make musical notes issue from the rear of their anatomy, so that you would think they were singing. . . . Human organs, without the excitement of lust, could have obeyed [the] human will for all the purposes of parenthood. . . . At a time when there was no unruly lust to excite the organs of generation and when all that was needed was done by deliberate choice, the seminal flow could have

reached the womb with as little rupture of the hymen and by the same vaginal ducts as is at present the case, in reverse, with the menstrual flux. . . . Perhaps these matters are somewhat too delicate for further discussion.

As one has seen, delicacy was seldom a problem for the early Christian fathers. Augustine's hesitation to continue with his ducts, fluxes, and flows probably came from a realization that if semen didn't break the hymen surely the birth of a child would, so up the chimney goes virginal vaginal intercourse.

Original sin damned a soul to Limbo, a no-man's land for unchristened Christians, *unless* saved by the blessed sacrament Baptism. Fornication damned a soul to eternal hell.

Fortunately, it took till medieval times for all these damned Christians to find out what they were headed for. As it took theologians centuries to catalogue all the sins of humanity, and sexuality, logic tells us it would take them a few more centuries to raise hell.

Let's all be grateful *A History of Christianity* has researched Hell for us—it's a hell of a job:

> The three most influential medieval teachers, Augustine, Peter Lombard and Aquinas, all insisted that the pains of Hell were physical as well as mental and spiritual, and that real fire played a part in them. The general theory was that Hell included any horrible pain that the human imagination could conceive of, plus an infinite variety of others. . . . And that Jerome said that Hell was like a huge winepress. . . . Augustine said it was peopled by ferocious flesh-eating animals, which tore humans to bits slowly and painfully and were themselves undamaged by fire . . . [another theologian] . . . that the damned eat and tear their own flesh, and drink the gall of dragons and the venom of wasps, and suck the head of adders . . . [and another] . . . the

damned would be nourished with green bread, washed down with a mere cupful of stinking water . . . [and one more claimed] . . . that a hundred million damned souls would be squeezed into every square mile of Hell and would thus be treated "like grapes in a press, bricks in a furnace, salt sediment in a barrel of pickled fish, and sheep in a slaughterhouse."

Don't go away, there's more: the layered-look Hell designed by the poet Dante which Will Durant describes as ". . . dark and frightening abysses between gigantic murky rocks; steaming, stinking marshes, torrents, lakes and streams; storms of rain, snow, hail, and brands of fire; blood-stilling shrieks and groans." This describes Hell divinely but only angels get to laugh.

After the fall of the Roman Empire and the end of the Classical Age, most of Europe entered the Dark Ages. The reasons for this drab period (c. 500 A.D. to 1000 A.D.) included the decay of governments, education, and urban existence, combined with frequent wars and an increase in barbaric clans (sound familiar?). This age was followed by the early medieval era, and with it a new phase in the history of sexual abstinence—courtly love, which introduced a radical change in attitudes between the sexes. Women were taken out of the pits and placed on pinnacles through a novel concept—romance. And even more novel was the *joyous* abstinence from sexual intercourse by noble males.

Courtly love first appeared during the late eleventh century in southern France at the court of Eleanor of Aquitaine, renowned for her political daring and independent thinking. She was a rare light for those emerging from the Dark—a patron of the arts, also the mother of Richard the Lion-Hearted, and twice a queen by marriage, first to the king of France and then to the king of England. Eleanor sponsored a new art form, troubadour poetry, which some historians claim originated in the courts of the sultans in the Orient. It eulogized the honor, happiness, and love which came in the service and devotion to a noble lady.

By the middle of the twelfth century the troubadours' songs and poetry could be heard in most of the courts of Europe and their poetic words had blossomed into feats of bravery and chivalrous deeds dedicated to noble ladies by courtly knights.

A thirteenth-century autobiography, *Frauendienst* (the service of women), by Ulrich von Lichtenstein gives a scenario—better termed a harrowing portrait—of a courtly love "affair" between a devoted knight and a noble lady, who accepted his services without granting her "favors."

At twelve Ulrich fell for a princess who had all the necessary requirements for a chivalrous affair—a noble birth higher than his, older than he, rich, married and arrogant enough to accept a love slave. The next five years Ulrich practiced, secretly, the rules of courtly love: deep sighs; a poor appetite; wistful glances; inward trembling; and sleepless nights. During this time Ulrich's only happiness was stealing his princess' bath water and reverently drinking it.

After thirteen years of stouthearted service to his noble lady, Ulrich celebrated with the gift of one of his fingers, which he claimed was lost lancing in her service—actually he had it sliced off by a friend. His princess was touched, enough to say she would glance upon it daily, but not touched enough to relinquish a "favor" (the honor of carrying her ribbon or a chaste kiss).

In desperation Ulrich devised a bizarre, incredible feat. He challenged to lance every knight between Venice and Bohemia attired as the goddess Venus. After this whacky announcement Ulrich gathered together a retinue of squires, musicians, and maids-in-waiting worthy of a love goddess, then left for Venice to do some shopping. He first purchased twelve white gowns custom made for his girth. Then a wig which dangled two braids that hung to his waist and were laced with pearls. Then came a heady purchase of a jeweled tiara and veil. Thus attired this heavenly vision, in five weeks, completed his feat—lancing eight tournaments a day and amassing 307 broken lances from his opponents. His only respite in these battle-weary weeks was a brief visit with his wife and children.

In the twelfth century, Europe suffered a gradual collapse of the feudal system balanced by a corresponding growth in educational institutions and urban areas. These advances into the Renaissance shifted the human perspective. As man began to perceive the complexity of his universe, he sought solutions in scientific theories, rather than in gods and duty. In a small way, courtly love was a last hurrah for unified Christian attitudes on sexuality.

The spearhead for religious reformation was the German monk Martin Luther. He questioned two great supremacies: the supreme power of the papacy and the goodness of a God that would damn lowly humans for uncontrollable weaknesses. *The Natural History of Love* says:

> Luther found in sex an ideal weapon in his war against Rome. He early sanctioned marriage of priests and hotly argued that celibacy had been invented by the Devil as a source of sin; . . . and still later in life (1532) he held that Christ had probably committed adultery with Mary Magdalene and other women so as to partake fully of the nature of men.

Luther had a popular cause when he questioned corruption in the Vatican, since the Church had condoned a debasement of the papacy during the nefarious reign (1492 to 1503) of the Borgia pope, Alexander VI.

The Church knew what it was buying—though selling is possibly more accurate—as it is rumored Rodrigo Borgia bought the papacy in an auction among the cardinals.

As vice (apt!) chancellor to the pope, Borgia flaunted his disregard of twelfth-century rulings that the clergy remain celibate. True, he never married, but he had a score of mistresses, concubines, and illegitimate children. And two of his issue, Lucrezia and Cesare, speedily assisted their father the pope to become infamous throughout Italy and all of Europe. Shortly after his coronation, reports began appearing that Alexander, in his sixties, was having incestous relations with his daughter, Lucrezia, and that his son Cesare was his sexual rival. And after Lucrezia bore a child out of these incestous acts, there appeared two papal bulls. The first recognized the child as the illegitimate son of Cesare; the second proclaimed Alexander his father. Which goes to prove not all popes are infallible on certain issues.

In 1532, John Calvin, a student of theology and law in Paris, joined the Reform movement and aligned himself closely to Luther's condemnation of celibacy for the clergy. He believed the celibate state was not in everyone's power. And while sexual intercourse had previously been considered a "pollutant," God himself must not have found it so, for he chose it as a method for procreation. His religion, Calvinism (which later, in England and America, became the basis for the Puritan faith), encouraged the enjoyment of sex in marriage. So positive was Calvin that sex was not a sin, his religion granted divorces to wives with impotent husbands. Not since the ancient Judaic faith had sexual intercourse, in the Western world, received such affirmation for those married.

Finally, after fifteen centuries, the celibate state was out of date.

Agreed, there are to this day in both Western and Eastern cultures celibate communities, both religious and non. But with an increase in population, they get proportionately smaller and often fizzle. A qualified example is the Shaker movement in America, which was founded in the late eighteenth century. By 1840 there were Shaker communities in eight states with a total membership of six thousand. In 1905 membership was down to one thousand and by the mid-twentieth century the Shakers were almost nonexistent.

The Shakers acquired their quirky name from a dance they performed every night before retiring. In it, they coeducationally whirled, shook, sang, and shouted. And *The New Celibacy* adds:

> Most interpreters of this "whirling" activity see it as a technique the Shakers used to "neutralize the desire for coition" or as a release from sexual tension. The "dance" is also often considered to be orgasmic—a form of communal sex growing from the renunciation of genital sex.

As an ideal, the celibate state may have received its final blow scientifically. In the early 1900s Sigmund Freud claimed sublimation of the sexual drive (not a conscious process) produces neuroses or disorders in those "who are trying to be better than their constitution permits them to be." And Freud went even further, saying:

> . . . that the conflict from this powerful impulse [sex] brings out all the ethical and aesthetic forces in the psychic life and "steels" the character: and this is undoubtedly true by some specially favored individuals. . . . But in by far the largest number of cases the struggle against one's sexuality consumes the individual's energy at the very same time when the young man needs all his powers to establish his place and station in the world. . . . In general my impression is that sexual abstinence does not promote the development of energetic, independent men of action, original thinkers or bold innovators and reformers; far more frequently it develops well-behaved weaklings who are subsequently lost in the great multitude . . .

So much for abstinence.

8

CASTRATION COMPLEXITY

I saw the mosques, the seraglio, Santa Sophia. In the seraglio, a dwarf, the sultan's dwarf, was playing with white eunuchs outside the throne room; the dwarf was hideous, expensively dressed in European style—gaiters, overcoat, watch chain. As for the eunuchs . . . I wasn't prepared for them. They looked like nasty old women. The sight of them makes you nervous, and torments the imagination. You find yourself devoured by curiosity, and at the same time the bourgeois in you makes you loathe them. The anti-normality of their appearance is a shock to one's virility. Explain that to me. No question, though, that they are one of the most curious products of the human hand. What wouldn't I have given, in the Orient, to become a friend of a eunuch!

This lyrical passage, a prejudicial description of a single genre in male castration, is from a letter Gustave Flaubert wrote while touring Istanbul in the mid-nineteenth century. Yet even today, there are misconceptions about degrees of castration, their physiological and psychological effects, and the history of eunuchs through the ages. Also, there is much erroneous information about the character and physical appearance of emasculated males.

Male castration has four degrees: the clean-shaven (penis and testicles removed), stoned (testicles removed), tailless (penis removed), and crushed balls (painfully self-explanatory).

And, contrary to indiscriminate beliefs, these castrated males are not necessarily: fat, tall, mean, pale, lazy, nasally repellent, gaudy dressers, sweets fanatics, effeminate, despondent forever, weak-minded, chaste in the head, haters of women and children, or inept at dancing, conversation, fencing, warfare, marine navigation, creativity, wooing, or incapable of doing it.

Castration of males has a four-millennium history, having been done by religious fanatics, conquering warlords, suspicious sultans, knife-neurotic jurists, below-the-navel plastic surgeons, German mines, women with poor and good aim, slave dealers, vacuum cleaner fans, careless carpenters, injudicious athletes, and creative self-surgeons.

Self-castration has an even longer history, for it is done by wild beasts (boars with leprous-type sores on their testicles will castrate themselves on a tree stump to get relief), frenzied members of ancient and not-so-ancient cults, and all-for-realism transsexuals in current society.

The origin of the word *eunuch* is Greek and means "the guardian of the bed." "Winner take all" would be historically more appropriate, for in ancient time triumphant armies or tribes would reduce their percentage of future attacks through the surgical sterilization of as many enemy males as they could lay their knives on. Castration was also inflicted for punishment and humiliation. Darius I, after crushing a revolt by Assyrians and Babylonians against his Persian rule, discriminatingly chose five hundred of the most handsome youths for genital severance. In all probability these lads were fated to become anal sex objects for his courtiers.

In Rome in 65 A.D., the Emperor Nero *legally* castrated a young lad, and then *legally* married him. Castration was illegal for a Roman citizen, due largely to a persistent decline in births by cynical Roman nobles. Nero's excuse to his government was that the lad closely resembled his recently deceased pregnant wife Poppaea—who, story had it, was murdered by a kick to the stomach from her loving husband.

Along with imperial clout, Romans were believers in religious clout—especially that of a lofty god or goddess. Therefore, in 204 B.C., when Hannibal almost had Roman armies backed to their walls, pragmatic Romans turned to the ancient Phrygian Mother of the Gods to save them. This meant importing from Asia Minor its stone idol (some claim phallic in design) and Cybele, its high priestess, who was attended by castrated males.

Every spring Cybele threw a four-day bash in honor of the Mother God and her symbol of fertility. The party was a paradox, for on the third day, the Day of Blood, the festivities included novitiate priests who, in a religious twit, castrated themselves, then flung their severed genitals on an altar consecrated to fertility. *The Golden Bough* gives us the Roman interpretation of this ancient rite:

> . . . at the beginning of the spring, when multitudes thronged to the sanctuary from Syria . . . the flutes played, the drums beat, and the eunuch priests slashed themselves with knives, the religious excitement spread like a wave among the crowd of onlookers, and many a one did that which he little thought to do when he came

as a holiday spectator to the festival. For man after man, his veins throbbing with the music, his eyes fascinated by the sight of the streaming blood, flung his garments from him, leaped forth with a shout, and seizing one of the swords which stood ready for the purpose, castrated himself on the spot. Then he ran through the city, holding the bloody pieces in his hand, till he threw them into one of the houses which he passed in his mad career. The household thus honored had to furnish him with a suit of female attire and female ornaments, which he wore the rest of his life.

Certain considerate historians have made lengthy lists to prove that eunuchs, down through time, had an equal chance—along with the rest of the human race—to suffer a brain strain or develop thick skin.

During these historians' research a mysterious item surfaced. *Curiosities of Erotic Physiology* reports there are ecclesiastical writers (unnamed) who declare Saint John the Apostle was a eunuch. Initially, this seems unlikely. Chiefly because it has, for centuries, remained such a well-kept secret. And it's even more suspect when one considers that Jews so despised damage to a male's genitals that Deuteronomy says: "He that is wounded in the stones, or hath his privy member cut off, shall not enter the congregation of the Lord." And Tannahill's *Sex in History* states that the Western Church inherited this view from the ancient Hebrews. Therefore, with these weighty prejudices, it seems unlikely that John "the Eunuch" would be chosen as not only a disciple but a "pillar" for the crusading—Judaic rostered—Christian faith.

Could it be that these nameless ecclesiastic writers were misled by John being portrayed, into medieval time in the West, as the only beardless apostle in an age of bewhiskered males? Perhaps the Byzantine artists who depicted John as an aging man with a long white beard were more informed, since John lived a long life and died, at the age of ninety, not far from Byzantium (Istanbul). Though, it would be realistic for John to be beardless at the time of the Last Supper, for he was only twenty when Jesus died.

Still, before we scratch John from the eunuch slate, there is the unsolved mystery: Why did Jesus choose John, above all other apostles, as the Beloved Disciple who "shall not taste death" until he was once again in the sight of the Lord? Why did John require—or deserve—a special entrée to the Messianic kingdom? Could it be that Jesus was giving John the protection and preferential treatment he gave to earthy prostitutes and other outcasts?

In the total history of castrated males, only a small percent have protected beds or the activities that might transpire on them; they generally seem interested in bigger things.

During the second-century-A.D. Han dynasty in China, for instance, eunuchs controlled a majority of the Imperial Court's influential positions and, to regain control of the government, the consort's families were forced to massacre all of them. But the prime example for individual eunuch power coupled with authoritative command came in the early fifteenth century, with the equivalent of a Christopher Columbus for the Orient. Eighty-seven years before Columbus set sail for the "East," the eunuch Cheng Ho set his sails for the Western Oceans. Cheng (his surname) had been castrated as a war trophy at the age of ten for the newly established Ming dynasty, when they reclaimed the Yunnan province from the Mongols. After capture, Cheng worked his way up from a young orderly in the Chinese army to a court eunuch with an Imperial crown contact. In 1405, at the age of thirty-four, Cheng was appointed by his emperor commander in chief of a naval armada consisting of three hundred ships and twenty-seven thousand men—impressive, considering that the *Santa María* was manned by thirty-nine men, the *Pinta*, by twenty-six, and the *Nina*, by twenty-two.

In the next twenty-seven years, Cheng made a total of seven voyages. He traveled as far as Java in the South China Seas, sailed up both coasts of India, took a swing through the Persian Gulf, went to the neck of the Red Sea, and sailed down the east African coast. Besides being an explorer Cheng was a diplomatic agent for Imperial China, bringing back envoys from thirty states to pay homage to his emperor.

In Italy, during the sixteenth century, eunuchs were far from outcasts in the Roman Catholic Church. Their popularity was due to a unique job opportunity created by a new art form—opera—and a revolutionary new style in singing, bel canto ("beautiful song"), characterized by a clarity of tone combined with brilliant vocal displays that were mastered only after years of training. But these skills created a sexist quandry, as there was no one to sing the soprano's refrains. For centuries the Church and Catholic Europe followed Saint Paul's injunction, "Let your women keep silence in the churches." Therefore, women were banned from performing not only in church rituals but all stage productions. The solution lay in making a man for the job, but to do so underhandedly, since castration was prohibited by Church law.

Singled out for emasculation were exceptional choirboys between the ages of six and seven. After recovery from his operation, the boy would continue taking voice lessons until he developed "an extraordinary chest expansion, an exemplary use of diaphragm to support and control the emission of breath, an agile supple throat, great virtuosity and imagination in vocal display and ornamentation, and, in a majority of cases, a notable degree of personal vanity" (Encyclopaedia Britannica).

There is little doubt that these adult male sopranos became the first prima donnas of their time—celebrated and adored by all music lovers and courted by the luminaries of the age. Emperor Napoleon Bonaparte invited a famed castrato to entertain his Parisian court, and Philip V of Spain signed another on as his resident court singer. In the 1740s the castrati system came close to altering the history of music when composer Franz Joseph Haydn, father of the symphony and the string quartet, was selected for castration by his Viennese choirmaster. Only Haydn's parents' refusal to sanction his operation saved him.

The medical journal *Urology* gives us a joyous ending to this tragic operatic arrangement. After extensive research into the histories of thousands of males castrated for church choirs and opera companies, M. M. Melicow reports that they had active love lives, including heterosexual love affairs and successful, though childless, marriages.

Legally, though, many religions resist marriage for eunuchs. For instance, the Roman Catholic Church (along with other faiths) bans impotent men from marriage. As recently as 1982 a young American paraplegic was denied the right to marry in the Church unless he had a doctor's statement confirming he could consummate his marriage. The man's doctor refused, claiming uncertainty. Fortunately, a kindly bishop altered the church's position after proving no medical specialist, or church official, could pronounce the young man permanently impotent.

Through the ages castration appears to have broken through most cultural and color barriers (sex too—for females have a similar sad history). Take those haunting white eunuchs espied in the sultan's palace by Flaubert. During the fifteenth century young men and boys were exported to the sultans of the East from Germany, Russia, and the Slavic countries. They were sold as slaves to these Moslem rulers for their personal servants and guards. White eunuchs were preferred for palace security, because they were politically powerless in a Moslem culture. Also, with the stigma of castration, it was believed a eunuch's loyalty would remain, by necessity, constant to his foreign master.

The penis of the white eunuch remained permanently attached. It was a symbol in the East (and most points West) of male aggression combined with strength and athletic agility. Because of this, the white eunuch was banned from the harem. Sultans in the Orient knew all the ins and outs, and had been aware since Roman time that eunuchs were popular sex partners among jaded married ladies. Many a Roman matron had discovered a partially emasculated male was far from impotent but *always* sterile.

White eunuchs were seldom castrated before puberty to prevent their developing all the manifestations of those born eunuchs—namely, a tiny penis, incomplete muscular development, high-pitched voice, lack of body hair, gaunt stature, tendency to fatigue, sallow complexion, and no beard, but a full head of hair.

The youthful Flaubert's merciless label of "nasty old women" was perhaps inspired by his admitted prejudice or just a reaction to his first sight of white males past their prime dressed in foreign, flamboyant—almost female—attire. Then again, these eunuchs might have been effeminate homosexuals; among castrated males are both heterosexuals and gays. If they keep their pants on, most male eunuchs will "pass" as *all* boy, if castrated after puberty.

The black eunuch imported by these same sultans has another history entirely. These castrated males come from many areas of Africa to serve as guards and servants in the harems of Moslem rulers. The black eunuch was always clean-shaven—minus everything—and if ugly, so much the better, for a slave dealer's price would go up and resale along with it. Clean-shaven eunuchs never went cheap. They were far too rare. Researchers claim a survival rate of only one-fourth for the Negro boys who were operated on between the ages of eight and ten for the removal of penis and testes. If castration was performed after fifteen years of age, the death rate could almost triple.

Clean-shaven eunuchs who did survive urinated through

a quill, and their sexual interchange was limited to anal or oral eroticism. But, whether clean-shaven or stoned, boys castrated before puberty usually suffered a permanent major decrease in libido (sexual interest and drive).

In some cases this could be a blessing, as the eighteenth-century political philosopher Montesquieu describes in the *Persian Letters* the sexual frustrations of a eunuch fully castrated as an adult:

> When my master first determined to entrust his women to me, and induced me by a thousand promises, supported by as many threats, to part with myself forever, almost wearied out with painful service, I resolved to sacrifice my passions to my tranquility and fortune.
>
> Wretch that I was . . . I flattered myself with the gain, but did not consider the loss. I hoped to be delivered from the assaults of love, by the incapability of satisfying it. Alas! the effect of the passions were destroyed in me, without extinguishing the cause; and very far from feeling relieved, I found myself surrounded with objects by which these passions were more and more irritated. I entered the harem, where all I saw excited my regret for the loss I had sustained; every minute offered excitement to desire. Numberless charms seemed to present themselves before me, only to rive my heart with despair. To complete my misfortune, I had ever before my eyes the happy possessor of all these charms. . . . I have never conducted a lady to my master's bed, and assisted in undressing her, than I returned to my chamber, with my heart bursting with rage, envy and despair . . . one day as I was helping one of the ladies into the bath . . . I dared to place my hand upon the most formidable spot upon a woman. Upon recovering myself, I made sure of that day's being the last of my life. I was fortunate enough, however, to escape with my life. . . .

This intelligent, sensitive analysis of a perpetual Catch-22 situation should eliminate forever the misconception that eunuchs are fated to be dull-witted, sexless numbskulls.

Sexual Variance describes a Hindu sect in India whose members are self-castrated males dedicated to a mono-penis—that of the Godhead, Krishna. These males consider their bodies passive agents for this diety's sexual gratification. Besides wearing female attire, they adopt feminine habits, movements, and behavior, including the imitation of menstruation.

Hinduism is one of the few ancient and modern religions in this world to sanctify both physical and mental sexuality. And this enlightened spirit does not exclude the sexuality of eunuchs. Hinduism defines the eunuch as the third sex of which there are four categories: "the waterless," or male eunuchs whose testicles have dried up; "testicles voided," castrated males; "the neuter," hermaphrodites; and "not women," castrated females. The third sex has one basic natural function, to provide alternative techniques for sexual gratification.

Though not considered religious sects, there are in India and in Pakistan communities of castrated males who prostitute themselves as passive female agents. They are called Hijras and consider themselves skilled, not only in sexual diversions but as trained musicians and dancers. Young boys taken into these communities were castrated or had their organs crushed during infancy until they had wasted away. *The Encyclopedia of Sexual Behavior* says a passive entrance is created in these youths by the repeated insertion of greased gradated wooden or metal cones into their rectums until the opening could easily admit three fingers. All members wear female clothing, have feminine names, and assume girlish manners and gestures. Genetic females are strictly taboo, but hermaphrodites who accept the Hijra code of living are allowed membership.

What was done, you ask, with all these castrated genitals? Well, most Chinese carried their pickled testicles in jars that hung around their necks. In other areas eunuchs chose to have their preserved genitals buried with them.

Some chose to make them altar offerings, mantle decorations, or gifts for special occasions. Many were tossed away as worthless tokens. And, in the last decade or so, through the miracle of modern medicine, some dismembered penises have become vaginas.

In none of the aforementioned types of castration have emasculated males suffered severe cases of vagina envy. Only one category of castrated male suffers the horn of this dilemma—the male transsexual, whose "perversion" is inexplicable to most heterosexuals and homosexuals, both male and female.

Male transsexuals who go flat out for the castration of their penis and testicles are thought by most heterosexuals to be homosexuals who have lost their marbles, etc. This analysis is rejected by both transsexuals and homosexuals. The horror of damage to the penis, or the loss of it, is as great for the male homosexual as it is for the male heterosexual. Members of both groups consider the penis as a vital tool of lovemaking and a magnificent physical affirmation of maleness.

In contrast, the male transsexual so despises his organ that he will go to great expense and suffer extreme pain for the removal of his genitals and the extermination of every aspect of his maleness.

There appears the occasional off-again-on-again transsexual who regrets, too late, the voluntary forfeiture of his sexual organ, but this is rare. Most appear to share the conviction that, since early childhood, they have been "females trapped within male bodies." Gender identity is never an inner problem for the transsexual; it's his exterior that's not what it ought to be.

In most cases, the first step a transsexual takes to alter his exterior is chemical castration through massive doses of estrogen, which result in impotence and shrinkage of the testicles. Taken over a long period of time, this hormone also decreases libido, increases the size of the breasts and buttocks, and alters neck, shoulders, and wrists to feminine size and proportion. It even replaces muscle sinew with fatty deposits in the legs and arms, including the armpits, with a corresponding loss of physical strength. To retain these feminine characteristics, male transsexuals will continue estrogen therapy for the rest of their lives, despite the increased risk of cancer of the breast. The hormone does not affect vocal range or decrease facial or body hair. Voice and hair alterations often are achieved through lengthy and costly visits to voice therapists and hair-removal clinics. Any tendency toward baldness is corrected by hair transplants or by wigs. Also, the male's Adam's apple is usually more prominent than the female's, so many transsexuals choose to have this surgically "shaved." And, some who are dissatisfied with the estrogen enlargement of their breasts, buttocks, and hips favor silicone injections or implants in one or all of these parts. Also, before any surgery is performed, a reputable physician will require extensive psychiatric evaluation of his patient and up to a year of "successful" living as a female, whatever that means.

Of course, all of this takes mucho bucks and guts. Neither of which were needed before 1952, since previous to then no surgeon in the world could *legally* perform a sex transference operation. But in 1951 an ex-GI, George (Christine) Jorgensen, went to Denmark and convinced a German surgeon the only solution for a male transsexual was total castration. This took a bit of doing, for medical science is hesitant to recognize the distinctive phenomenon of transsexuality. In addition, there is the battle against a surgeon's natural disinclination to perform any type of castration unless it is critical to a patient's survival.

When the news broke of Jorgensen's operation, many men around the world were revolted and women, this globe's first-rate second-class citizens, were dumbfounded.

But the real eye-opener for medical science came when Dr. Christian Hamburger, Jorgensen's surgeon, received over five hundred letters from people around the world, all pleading for similar surgery. From that day on the medical profession recognized castration as a vital procedure for many a male transsexual.

And what about the castrated penis that becomes a vagina? Does it really work? Does it look like a vagina—if you knew what one looked like? By any stroke of luck and pluck, does the clitoris function? Does it come with a built-in G spot?

Happy to say the answer is yes to all of the above—with the possible exception of the Graffenberg spot, which is a search for the Holy Grail in any vagina.

In the last few decades, as transsexuals alter their genitals, the following curious data have emerged:

1. No one knows for sure what causes transsexualism. We only know that it affects a minority of the world's population and only one child in a family; that this child is usually male; that his father is absent or emotionally uninterested in being a parent. Also, one psychiatric researcher found that nearly all of his male transsexual patients had mothers who admitted to gender identity ambivalence previous to their marriages.

2. In the Western world males requesting transference surgery outnumber females eight to one, yet in Eastern Europe there are more requests for female to male surgery than vice versa.

3. Psychotherapy, electroshock therapy, and drug therapy have all failed to alter a transsexual's belief in his or her gender identity. Male transsexuals claim that this is not surprising since they know they are females, and that just as a genetic female is incapable of altering her gender identity, so indeed is a male transsexual incapable of such an alteration in identity.

4. After castration, either surgical or chemical, male transsexuals are delighted with the decrease in their libido, because they believe it brings their sexual appetite more in line with the less intensive sex drive of a woman.

5. It is by no means rare for male transsexuals to be asexual; yet it is far from common in genetic males.

6. Castrated males rarely get gout (a disease in which ninety-five percent of the victims are male) or leprosy. In early times gout was considered the disease of lechery, and this old wives' tale probably has some truth in it. With increased libido, the blood level of male testosterone rises, and gout has an intriguing connection with this male hormone.

7. As young children, all male transsexuals preferred to be seated while urinating, and by adolescence this had not abated and was compounded by a developed pattern of cross-dressing, which never evoked sexual excitement (such as it does for transvestites) but created a sense of well-being and happiness.

8. While estrogen therapy had a calming effect on male transsexuals, the administration of the male sex hormone androgen has the opposite effect and, while it increases sexual drive, it has no effect in altering the character or direction of sexual urges.

9. After surgical transference, male transsexuals who do not marry are often tempted to take up prostitution, because they get pleasure from heterosexual males accepting them as sexy females and being willing to pay for their sex services.

10. A castrated penis is preferred for the creation of a vagina, because skin grafts from other areas of the body are likely to produce hair. Before insertion in the patient, the skin of the penis is stripped off and turned inside out like the finger of a glove. The tip end—the glans—becomes the roof of the vagina because inside out and upside down it is a remarkable lookalike for a genetic female's cervix. In fact, so

remarkable is this entire vagina, it has fooled more than one gynecologist. Some male transsexuals have even succeeded in passing the physical exam for the women's military service.

11. Well over ten percent of males denied sexual transference operations attempt self-castration, and many succeed.

Finally, what is the success rate for those who do receive transference surgically? Physically, it is highly successful because the vagina functions well and looks even better. But emotionally the picture is not so rosy. In 1976 this author interviewed a well-known London urologist (anonymous by preference) who, after a decade of sexual transference surgery, decided to retire from this type of surgical procedure. The urologist had discovered in follow-up examinations that there was a less than fifty percent increase in his patients' emotional well-being, and a number had attempted suicide.

The lack of realistic goals for some male transsexuals is one reason for the lower percentage in emotional adjustment. For example, surgeons have reported repeated demands for implantation of ovaries and uteri in order that they might become pregnant, a miracle still beyond medical science.

But one miracle was reported recently from Paris, when French surgeons announced that they had successfully reattached a young male's severed penis and testicles. The operation took twelve hours of delicate microsurgery. Previous to this, doctors had reported reattachment of penises, but never both penis and testicles. The operation was done in a hospital near Paris in April 1977 and not announced until physicians had determined it a complete success. The twenty-one-year old man had castrated himself in a violent schizophrenic crisis. The head surgeon reported that after the surgery, the patient was capable of a normal sex life, but was sterile.

Unfortunately, microsurgery was an unknown procedure when the Germans employed castration mines during World War II. These land mines, touched off by a mere footstep, were devised so that the first explosion hurled the mine to crotch level, and the second detonation was aimed for castration of the genitals. For the lucky soldier whose penis remained undamaged but who lost his testicles, the picture was not nearly so bleak as physicians predicted it would be, for in most cases the men were still able to engage in intercourse, and it was eventually discovered that these men were manufacturing testosterone from another source—the adrenal glands. Enough testosterone was produced to allow erections, orgasms, and ejaculations. This discovery set off in-depth studies on hormonal therapy for sexual rejuvenation and this has revived many a lapsed member, though most physicians still claim the best solution for most impotence can be found above the neck.

One type of castration has, as yet, not been defined. The category is "crushed balls" and it had, according to the father of medicine, Hippocrates, an ancient history and a curious origin. The learned doctor ascribed the cause for a preponderance of impotent, effeminate males, found in Scythian nomadic tribes, to extensive horseback riding. This is a provocative theory, because the Scythians were warriors who wandered between Central Asia and southern Russia, from the eighth to the fourth century B.C., using a new form of tactical warfare—the cavalry. Humans had been riding animals since 1300 B.C., but it was the Scythians who first mastered the art of horse riding and used it for large-scale conquests. So treasured was the horse in Scythian culture that after his death a tribal chieftain was buried in his cavernous tomb with as many steeds as his burial vault could hold. The bodies of horses were stacked one on top of another in several rooms with only a limited space reserved for the slain bodies of the chieftain's wife and favorite servants.

Scythians were the first to geld a horse, but the castration of animals dates as far back as 4000 B.C., when primitive farmers converted bulls to oxen so they would be easier to handle and so provide an additional source of nonhuman power.

In the whole history of castration the saddest to record are those who were forced to this sacrifice by social reformers to save society. Kinsey gives this succinct description of those unmercifully cut for the salvation of mankind:

> In more recent decades, both in Europe and this country, castrations have been rationalized as attempts to modify some aspect of the individual's sexual behavior: to stop masturbation, to transform homosexual into heterosexual patterns of behavior, to control exhibitionists and, in particular, to control adults who sexually "molest" children. Castrations have been used in both Europe and in this country to prevent feeble-minded, criminal or irresponsible individuals from becoming parents; but simple sterilization would satisfy that end. . . . Castrations have, of course, been necessarily performed when testes were diseased . . .

The bad news is that some of the above cases "humanely" included the removal of both testes and penis. The good news is that physical (subliminal has another Freudian history) castration for humans is disappearing.

9

MAN THE PUMP, THE PENIS IS INFLAMED

That drip—gonorrhea—has been around so long no one knows for sure when it made its first attack on the human penis. One ancient source, cuneiform writings from the sixth century B.C., describes the king of Assyria being treated by priests for a disease that has all the signs and symptoms of gonorrhea. Other records with similar descriptions date back to ancient China and Egypt. Some medical historians also believe this disease is depicted in the Bible and one reason the ancient Hebrews used the rite of circumcision was as a preventive measure against the transmission of what scientists now label V.D.G.

In 150 A.D., Galen, a

Greek physician to Roman emperors and gladiators, tagged the diseased mucus drip gonorrhea (the flow of seed). And the origin of *venereal* is a combination of Venus, the Roman goddess of love, plus *ery*, which gives us venery or lovemaking. From these origins we can assume the Roman Empire had something to be concerned about.

Since VD tends to increase during wartime and spreads along with conquests, the odds are that most barbaric clans and ancient communities were suffering from this sexually transmitted disease. One known exception on this globe is the kingdom of the beasts, since venereal disease appears to be a rarity in all wild species. Not so fortunate are domestic animals, especially those given artificial insemination. (Gonorrhea communicated by artificial insemination is not unknown in humans either.) It is presumed that animals in the wild are protected because the VD organisms are not in constant transmission (VD cells are short-lived or frail until they multiply in the protection of a body) due, in part, to harem-style mating and the female having a briefer sexual time span.

How can one spot this vile drip? *The Encyclopedia of Sexual Behavior* leaks some data to hotheaded males on how to recognize this particular STD (sexually transmitted disease):

> This most striking feature is a creamy, greenish-yellow discharge from the penis. This occurs after an incubation period of from two to seven days following sexual intercourse. . . . The discharge is sometimes asymptomatic, but usually it is accompanied by burning on urination, most often at the tip of the penis, which is somewhat red and swollen.

This tome goes on to say that if the disease goes untreated, complications could lead to a pile of bad news, such as the swelling of the testes to the size of an orange and/or the spread of the disease to the rectum (the disease can also be transmitted by anal intercourse—a common occurrence among male homosexuals). It also adds the fact that gonorrhea cannot be caught from "dirty" toilet seats, "dirty" towels, or muscular strain from overexercising.

Over the centuries, some of the euphemisms for gonorrhea have become symptomatically descriptive while others, perhaps to be expected with such an "intimate" disease, sound like friendly nicknames. Some are: a dose; a stain; the glue; a delicate taint; piss, pins, and needles; the gleet; a tear; a lulu; the burner; piss of pure cream; a hat and a cap; a horse and a trap; the gentleman's complaint; the clap (origin of clap is to embrace); and old joe.

These friendly nicknames could also point up the fact that, for many centuries, many men took the disease as a laughing matter. The laughter usually came from two different causes. In some cases this disease's symptoms would mysteriously disappear. Some of these cases were legitimate cures, but other sufferers only became asymptomatic, with gonorrhea becoming the origin of other serious diseases (such as crippling arthritis) which surfaced years later. Those who remained with symptoms often laughed, claiming that since there was no cure a tear was the price most males could expect to pay for an active, varied sex life.

After the discovery of antibiotics and a quick, cheap, and painless cure, most men began considering the clap (its most endearing nickname) a brief annoyance.

Just how large this number might be is clear if we consider that in the United States alone, the Public Health Service in December 1974 estimated this country had 2½ million cases annually. Over the world the estimate was 150 million cases.

In the United States there is an "in season" for gonorrhea—July and August (what a vacation!)—with the highest incidence coming from the Southern and Pacific Coast states. A 1981 survey in *The American Journal of Public Health* found that of 4,212 homosexual males, thirty-eight percent had contracted gonorrhea. (Sixty percent of 3,696 of these males said they had had at least one sexually transmitted disease.)

In 1981 the American news media pounced on a new strain of this disease which they hailed as "super-gonorrhea" (the official term is PPNG—penicillinase-producing *Neisseria gonorrhoeae*). This strain produces an enzyme that, though resistant to penicillin, is highly curable by other types of antibiotics.

From 1979 through the first nine months of 1981 the number of cases of "super-gonorrhea" in New York City jumped from 328 to 1,981 (strangely, they stopped counting after the cases numbered the same as the year). The city's health inspectors sought the cooperation of madams and prostitutes in forty of the city's brothels. Testing showed that forty percent of the prostitutes either had the disease or were carriers. The health department said they were not reporting these cases to the police, and the police said they had no intention of pressing the health authorities for information because of the importance of getting this "super" strain under control.

Dose for dose, gonorrhea has nowhere near the malignant history of that total rotter, syphilis. Before antibiotics, this disease killed or inflicted serious permanent disabilities on 25 percent of the unfortunates who became infected. The vile canker of syphilis broke out in epidemic proportions in Naples almost five hundred years ago. In 1494, the French king Charles VIII conquered the southern port with an army of men consisting mainly of mercenary bands gathered from many areas of Europe. Garrisoned within the city for several months, this unruly lot raped and whored their time away. But their sporting days were limited. Suddenly the ecstasies of Venus became suspect when tumors began to appear on their genitals. Even more alarming, as these tumors vanished, odious lesions began to attack, not only the genitals, but other parts of their bodies, including the mouth, lips, and eyes.

Neopolitans began screaming their sore spots were inflicted by the conquerors and tagging it "the French sickness." The French drew in their horns, claiming they had been poxed by "the Neopolitan disease."

When the French troops were withdrawn from Naples in 1495 and the infected mercenaries returned to their homelands, "the French sickness" spread throughout Europe. By 1505, a syphilitic plague had swept Europe and spread as far as the Middle East, India, and China. On its travels, the sickness became known as the enemy-nation-of-your-choice disease. The Egyptians called it the Syrian disease, the Russians blamed the Poles, the Chinese said it was the Portuguese, the Dutch bet it was Spanish, and the Turks took odds on the Christians. Naturally, all of the accused said vice was versa.

Today medical historians favor an early-sixteenth-century theory that claims syphilis was brought to Europe from the New World by sailors who manned Columbus's ships on his first voyage in 1492. This theory was backed by two sources, one a biography of Columbus written by his son Ferdinand, who wrote that on Columbus's return to Española (Haiti) in 1498 he found one out of four men left behind to establish a colony were dead or suffering from the plague that was devastating Europe. This sorry finding could indicate Columbus's crew had carried syphilis from Europe to the New World, but Ferdinand went on to write that a Spanish friar, left behind to compile a history of the Indians, said the disease had been known by the Indians for centuries and was described in their ancient legends.

Because it has the punch of a firsthand account the second source is even more convincing. In 1539 a physician,

Ruy Diaz de Isla, published a book in which he claimed to have treated some of Columbus's crewmen on their return from the New World for an unknown disease which he labeled *Morbo Serpentino* (the snake disease) because it became a hideous, creeping malady. The physician said the event occurred in 1493 in Barcelona. Additional research has confirmed the existence in Spain of a vile new disease that initially attacked the genital area. The illness was blamed not on sex but on the ominous alignment of the planets that occurred during the outbreak. This weird heavenly disease was called the Scorpio Epidemic because the planets Jupiter, Saturn, and Venus were in a rare line-up in the astrological sign Scorpio.

Although some question arises as to why it took the Barcelona physician over forty years to publish his story, few historians question its veracity. De Isla had a reputation for outstanding medical practice and is recognized by some as the discoverer of a first "cure" for syphilis, having noticed that a raging fever would arrest this dread disease.

By 1497, the disease was so prevalent in Paris that the French parliament panicked and ordered all those afflicted with the "large pox" to leave the city till cured. The government even allowed the evacuees a traveling allowance. Those too ill to travel were isolated in a home and left to the mercy of quacks, since legitimate physicians refused to treat the vile malady. In 1505, after it was determined the disease was contagious only (almost) through sexual intercourse, the afflicted were left to die in pain and shame on the streets of "the city of light."

A History of Prostitution written at the turn of this century by William Sanger, M.D., gives a humane although statistical look at the devastation wrought by syphilis during four centuries in Europe and America. He tells us that not till 1614 was a hospital opened for the care of the syphilitic patient. Then sufferers fortunate enough to gain entrance were whipped on admittance and on release, as punishment for contracting the disease. This sadistic act continued until 1700.

Sanger also describes an eighteenth-century "hospital" for the syphilitic only, a pit of degradation and filth where patients slept six to a bed, in shifts of two. The patients were served only cheap broth and cheese, given dirty rags for bedding, took no baths, had their windows nailed shut, and received little medicine and less treatment.

For the afflicted who survived into the nineteenth century, more humane conditions existed. Indeed, these improvements must have had quite an impact. Several patients soon discovered there was life in the old boy yet, since Sanger records that one coed hospital for syphilitic patients was forced to close their female wards after males began to party with the prostitutes down the hall. In fact, some syphilitic patients who were not in the latent stage of the disease claimed syphilis made them horny.

With better treatment and education on prevention, syphilis began to diminish by the end of the nineteenth century. Still, Sanger estimated that in the late nineteenth century a minimum of seventy-four thousand new cases appeared in New York annually. If each person suffered only one attack per year, this represented one sixth of the population over fifteen years of age.

Appropriately, one of the most vivid descriptions of this disease was given by the sixteenth-century Italian physician and poet who coined the word *syphilis*. Girolamo Fracastoro painted a grotesque portrait—especially for those of us who peep at syphilis over our twentieth-century shield of antibiotics. You might want to skip this:

> Most of them [syphilitics] had chancres upon the organs of generation. These chancres were obstinate; when cured in one place they reappeared in another, and the

work was never ended. Pustules with a hard surface appeared upon the skin, generally on the head [of the penis] first. On first appearing they were small, but gradually increased to the size of an acorn, which they resembled in shape. In some places they were dry, in others humid; some were livid, others white and pale, others again hard and reddish. They burst after a few days, and discharged an incredible quantity of vile fetid humor. When they began to suppurate they became true phagedaenic ulcers, consuming both flesh and bone. When they attacked the upper part of the body, they gave rise to malign fluxions, which gnawed the palate or the windpipe, or the throat, or the tonsils. Some patients lost their lips, others the nose, others the eyes, others the whole organs of generation. Many were troubled with moist tumors on the limbs, which grew as large as eggs or small loaves. When they burst, a white mucilaginous liquor exuded from them. . . . And if this were not enough, the patients suffered terrible pains . . . were languid, had no appetite, desired to remain constantly in bed.

Besides being an observant physician, Fracastoro was a poet of some repute. In 1530, in a poem written in the classical style of the day, he tells the tale of a swine shepherd named Syphilis who, angered when his herd was killed off in a drought that struck Española, rebelled against the gods. In revenge, the sun god Sirus struck Syphilis down with a new and virulent disease. Soon Europe adopted this legendary victim's name as the official term for the scourge that was ravaging their continent. The word *syphilis* possibly comes from the Greek words meaning *swine* and *love*. Note also, this poem proves the early acceptance that syphilis originated in the New World, and the choice of swine to stress filth.

In 1530, Nuremberg physician and alchemist Paracelsus, the first to replace vegetable remedies with chemical drugs in medical science, discovered that carefully measured doses of mercury compounds cured syphilis if the disease had not reached the latent stage, which usually appeared about ten years after the earlier symptoms had subsided. Mercury was rubbed on or put in plasters and applied to the lesions. It was also swallowed in pills and liquid doses, which could be very chancy, because mercury is highly poisonous and hard on the kidneys.

For over three decades, the only "cure" available had been a concoction a witch doctor—or a quack—would prescribe, the use of "holy wood," *guiacum*, imported from the West Indies. Many concoctions were made from the holy wood. Since syphilis was believed to have originated in the New World, and the Indians there appeared to have the disease in a milder form, many became convinced that this wood possessed miraculous qualities. Naturally, with the high cost of importation and the greed of quacks, the price was so high that only the wealthy could afford a "holy" cure. A tad sad were those forced to use homemade remedies such as sassafras, sarsaparilla, or China root. Those less fortunate also tried "a hell of a cure"—taking a bumpy penis to a barber surgeon and having it cauterized with red-hot irons.

Wealthy or poor, famous or not, syphilis struck regardless of class. Besides the common man and the lowly peasant, the following list gives a glimpse of how widespread this disease was among the famous who ignited and flamed the history of the West for centuries:

Royalty: Charles VIII, Peter the Great, Henry VIII, Philip II, Francis I, Napoleon, Lord Randolph Churchill, and Benito Mussolini.

Explorers: Christopher Columbus (poetic justice!), Ferdinand Magellan, and Captain James Cook.

Composers: Hugo Wolf, Gaetano Donizetti, Ludwig van Beethoven, and Robert Schumann.

Artists: Benvenuto Cellini, Paul Gauguin, Francisco José de Goya, and Henri de Toulouse-Lautrec.

Writers: John Keats, the Marquis de Sade, Johann Wolf-

gang von Goethe, Charles-Pierre Baudelaire, Arthur Schopenhauer, Friedrich Wilhelm Nietzsche, Alexandre Dumas,
Guy de Maupassant, Stendhal, James Joyce, Oscar Wilde,
and Paul Verlaine.

Military Heroes: Cesare Borgia, George Custer, and
"Wild Bill" Hickok.

Gangster: "Scarface" (a nickname many a syphilitic
might have been tagged) Al Capone.

Clergy: Pope Julius II (who, thank the Lord, refused to
offer his foot for the kiss of homage after his toe rotted away
from syphilis) and priest Erasmus.

But euphemisms for syphilis were definitely class-con-
scious. The wealthy called it "the gentleman's disease,"
"blood disease," or "Venus's curse." Lower classes cursed
and called it "the crud" or "the pits."

There were no preventatives, other than celibacy, for
gonorrhea or syphilis until the middle of the sixteenth century. Well, actually, there was one—the purchase of a virgin
in a reputable house of prostitution. The first medical preventative was invented by Gabriel Fallopius (also the discoverer of the functions of some female tubing named after
him). Fallopius's device for prevention of venereal disease
was described in his book *De Morbo Gallico.* It's a slip of a
thing and goes like this:

> As often as a male has intercourse, he should if conve-
> nient wash his genitals and wipe them with a cloth. Af-
> terwards he should use a small linen cloth made to fit
> over the glans and draw forward the prepuce over the
> glans and if he can do so, it is well to moisten it with
> saliva or lotion. . . . If you fear *lest carries* [syphilis] . . .
> take the sheath of this linen cloth and place it in the
> canal [urethra]; I tried this experiment on eleven hun-
> dred men, and I call immortal God to witness not one of
> them was infected.

One would imagine with the publication of these odds,
in the midst of a raging epidemic, every stud in Europe

118

would be wearing little linen mittens when he entered the pits of passion. But the rub was these tacky mitts did not fit like a glove.

Linen mitts never became a hot item, having an awkward fit. But they were the primitive pattern for an upcoming sheath that did fit like a glove. This took another hundred years to evolve and was, supposedly, developed by an English army physician to Charles II. The king, a notorious womanizer, asked Dr./Colonel Condom to design a slick but secure cover for his "dart of love." The good doctor claimed the game was in the bag. The king was instructed to slip on, before sexual intercourse, the intestine of a lamb, calf, or goat and to secure it at the top with a snug little ribbon.

Mysteriously, Englishmen deny to this day the British discovery of the condom—the first nonmedicinal preventative for venereal disease. They even deny the existence of a Dr./Colonel Condom. But impossible to deny was the recorded fact that condoms were advertised for sale in several "speciality" shops during the mid-seventeenth century. Instead, the British gallantly insist the French take the honor for devising a preventative for "the French sickness." The British labeled the device "the French letter." One might imagine it would be labeled an envelope. At any rate, the French slammed back, calling it "the English overcoat."

The condom was given more practical nicknames as its popularity grew, both as a preventative for disease and a method of birth control. Some of these were: the armor, the safety cap, the potent ally, *THE* bag, the cabinet of love, the preserver, the shield, the amorial guise, the safety sheath, the machine, and the never-failing engine.

The condom, as a device to protect the penis from physical damage, stretches way back. It first popped up on a cave painting dating back to 15,000 B.C. in southern France (those cheers you hear are British). Way back then, cavemen certainly hadn't a clue about prevention of disease or contraception. Therefore, it is assumed the first sheath was a hot little number, made of animal hide, used to protect the penis from the cold and insect bites.

The cagiest ones were the ancient Egyptians (1350 B.C. to 12 B.C.), who had several different species of sheaths. Most were sturdy for the protection of the penis during battle. A lighter-weight sheath was worn daily to protect the penis from tropical skin diseases. Others were worn as narcissistic gadgets to advertise that the wearer had *some*thing on the balls. Some sheaths were adorned with jewels to define social status.

In the East, how-to-do-it manuals had the brass to admit their sheaths were worn by impotent males as dildos during lovemaking. They were made of precious metals or stones. Others were carved from horn, ivory, or wood. Still others were made of tin, lead, copper, or, on a really tough day, iron!

In the second century A.D., Roman author Antoninus Liberalis fittingly describes the Greek god Minos wearing a protective sheath because his semen was infested with serpents and scorpions. Some historians claim that Liberalis gave so accurate a description of Minos's use of a goat membrane, there was a good possibility that the studs of Imperial Rome were wrapping it up during sexual intercourse as a method of birth control—a theory given additional support by a dramatic decrease in the birthrate during the reign of Augustus, who deemed it a national emergency. But other historians demur, saying the use of the condom way back then for contraception is unlikely, since, other than Liberalis, no other source cited its use.

The condom began to appear in England during the eighteenth century as a shield against venereal disease. It was still, as in the seventeenth century, a gutsy intestine, but now the condom was softened by hours of soaking and then bathed in alkaline lye. Next, its muscular coat was exposed to the hellish vapor of burning brimstone, then scrubbed with soap and water, dried off, and blown up. The membrane was then filled with water and tested for leaks. If it passed muster, it was awarded a ribbon to shut its open mouth.

This scrupulous handwork made the early condom an expensive device. Not till 1839, when United States inventor Charles Goodyear accidently dropped rubber mixed with sulphur on a hot stove and stumbled upon vulcanization, was the condom cheaper by the dozen. The condom became cheaper yet after the invention of latex in 1930. In the Western world there has been little change in the condom since the 1930s.

In the East during the sixties the Japanese came out with a condom that was half again thinner, but it cannot be legally sold in the United States or in many other countries in the world. These nations claim this Japanese model is far too flimsy for their hardier members.

Many nations require condoms to measure up to other specifications before allowing entry. This is especially true when it comes to length. For instance, the condom in Britain is taller than those used by Yanks, and the Yanks' is taller than the Japanese. Surprisingly, the Yank is too tall for entry into Hungary and, staggeringly, the Hungarians are so shortsighted as to admit it.

Whatever the nation, condoms come in one of two materials: a gutsy, greasy intestine that clings or a rubbery jacket that comes either dry or wet.

In the Age of the Pill and antibiotics, are condoms in great demand today? You bet they are. One source makes the preposterous claim that three million condoms are produced daily around the world. After three centuries the condom still hangs in there. But even today in an age of open communication, the condom is still not allowed to be mentioned in ads on radio or TV, although the National Association of Broadcasters permits the promotion of remedies for jock itch, body lice, and hemorrhoids. Not to mention enemas, douches, tampons, and sanitary napkins.

This censorship seems particularly curious when we analyze the almost weekly reports in the media that despite antibiotics, venereal disease is on the increase and, in some areas, threatens to become a major epidemic if drastic measures are not taken.

One preventative available today is a questionable solution to conservative thinkers—antibiotic prophylaxis. This is especially true among physicians who fear that the abuse of wonder drugs might eventually bring on an immunity to their lifesaving benefits. In 1977 Dr. P. Frederick Sparling, head of the Division of Infectious Diseases, University of North Carolina, saw these additional dangers:

> Prophylactic use of oral antibiotics for persons possibly exposed to sexually transmitted disease is of uncertain efficiency in prevention of infection. Moreover, they may mask the initial signs and symptoms of infection, which would be particularly dangerous in the case of syphilis. Oral penicillin is known to be relatively ineffective in treatment of gonorrhea and might promote selection of resistant mutants. It is more reasonable at present to give therapy after the exposure, employing drugs and dosages adequate for treatment of gonorrhea and syphilis; this should be combined with adequate examination and cultures of the patient to establish a proper diagnosis if possible.

For another perspective on the use of antibiotic prophylaxis this author interviewed, in February 1983, Dr. Lonny Myers, a physician at the Cook County (Illinois) Department of Public Health for Sexually Transmitted Diseases. Dr. Myers says, "Gonorrhea is steadily increasing, and the main method used today to treat it—tracing contacts—absolutely does not work. Usually by the time the disease is diagnosed, at least one other person has been infected, since most persons who contract gonorrhea are sexually active. In addition to this, an increasing number of males are becoming asymptomatic—estimates go anywhere from fifteen to twenty-five percent. Therefore the disease travels faster than the treatment.

"Yet it has been known since the nineteen-forties that if you give someone small doses of antibiotics at the time of exposure to syphilis and gonorrhea, it brings the rate of incidence way, way down—by more than ninety percent, according to some studies. The reason for this is, at the time of transference, these organisms are just weak little fellows; therefore they can be easily destroyed by small doses of antibiotics. This information was published in *The Journal of the American Medical Association* in 1949. Antibiotic prophylaxis has been used in the armed services successfully over and over again. Yet to this day, it is not used for civilians.

"The use of prophylactic antibiotics in the control of sexually transmitted disease is verboten in the medical profession. There is no medical justification for this, since a person who has acne will be given a prescription for tetracycline over periods of years. A person with rheumatic fever could be on penicillin the rest of his life.

"Since World War I, even before the discovery of antibiotics as a cure for syphilis and gonorrhea, it has been known that a technique called postcoital disinfection was a highly effective preventive against disease. It's a simple procedure. Immediately after sexual intercourse, a male puts certain chemicals in an ointment on his penis. He puts the ointment on the outside of his penis to prevent syphilis and squirts it inside the urethra to prevent gonorrhea.

"Since the sixteenth century physicians have used huge doses of arsenic, bismuth, and mercury to treat syphilis *after* infection, when the organisms have invaded the body and multiplied. And like an army, the organisms capture and destroy one organ after another. Doctors who gave small doses of these same medicines for males to use immediately after intercourse were called quacks. The physicians who gave out huge—often dangerous—doses after infection were considered saviors and heroes. Absurd.

"And the same thing is happening today. The medical profession will give anyone all the antibiotics they need *after* they have contracted VD. We take care of you after the fact.

"And why? It boils down to one simple thing—our society is antisex outside of marriage. You cannot regulate that which you proscribe. So long as we tell people not to fuck, there is no way we are going to tell them how to do it responsibly. Still, we tell teenagers and others don't drink; but if you do drink, don't drive. Why aren't we saying: Don't fuck; but if you do, don't get diseased and don't get pregnant. We can't bring ourselves, in the case of teenagers, to accept the fact they are going to be sexually active in our society. Yet we beg them to be sexually active subliminally. You take these kids, whose hormone level is very high in terms of sex drive, and program them with sexy movies, TV shows, clothing, dances, and music. Then you tell them not to fuck. *And* we want them to do this from the age of eleven to twenty.

"It's a double message. No wonder people are confused. Sexiness is promoted as self-worth, but the physical expression of it is wrong. This is an irresponsible attitude for the medical profession—intelligent people trained and responsible for the physical and mental well-being of humans in our society.

"I wrote a letter to the AMA. It said, 'We've known how to prevent gonorrhea and syphilis since the sixteenth century—we now have, at least, some twenty other sexually transmitted diseases, some of which are very, very difficult to treat. Now if we use all the resources we have available as prevention for these two main diseases, we may well rid the world of gonorrhea and syphilis. And we win both ways. We demonstrate to the public how great the medical profession is—how we have rid the world of a scourge that has plagued mankind for five hundred years—*and* we still have eighteen diseases to fight chastity.'"

Dr. Myers has yet to receive a reply.

Methods for prevention of VD used by prostitutes around the world have been described by Edward M. Brecher, author of *The Sex Researchers*. In her forthcoming book on venereal disease, Dr. Myers advocates that those engaged in casual sex adopt similar measures. Mr. Brecher says most prostitutes use one or several of the following precautions—and all others should be taught:

> One very valuable measure is precoital "short-arm inspection" of the male genitals and surrounding area for [lesions], plus milking the urethra for exudate. Many prostitutes from Rome to Reno have for decades, perhaps centuries, performed this self-protecting ritual as conscientiously as do urologists. Precoital and postcoital soap-and-water washing of the male genitals, perhaps with a medicated soap, is also common, as is a postcoital douche or *bidet* for the female. Some American prostitutes thoroughly wash vulva and vagina with a soapy washcloth and warm water. Antibiotic prophylaxis is sometimes used either instead of or in addition to such topical measures. In the Far East, Penigen (a foaming vaginal tablet containing an antibiotic) is available and commonly used before coitus. Many Western European prostitutes (and a few in the U.S.) insist that the customer wear a condom. *There is no reason except prudery why such measures of self-protection cannot be taught to non-prostitutes*, female and male. The relative protection afforded by the common contraceptive creams, jellies, and foams against VD as well as pregnancy should also be widely publicized.

But, tragic to say, all of the above preventatives would prove futile in combating genital herpes, a highly contagious venereal disease approaching epidemic proportions today in the United States. This disease is not life-threatening (except in rare instances for females and newborns), but it is the scarlet pimple that strikes over fifty percent of its victims again—and again and again and again.

In August of 1981 the switchboard for the VD National Hotline received eleven thousand toll-free calls from around the country. The number-one concern of those seeking information was genital herpes. The second was gonorrhea. The fear of these two diseases, rarely life-threatening for males, comes despite a rise of 33.4 percent in syphilis cases from 1978 to 1980.

Because gonorrhea and syphilis are easily treatable and often preventable, most sexually active Yanks have focused their concern on a sexually transmitted disease that is incurable. Because herpes is a viral infection, any cure would involve messing around with the body's central nervous system—a route so complex it makes a trip to Saturn look like taking the A train.

The fear of an incurable disease and the shame of being one of those infected has many a man turning his back on the sexual revolution. A September 1982 Washington Post–ABC News poll found that of 1,505 unmarried people between the ages of eighteen and thirty-seven, fifty percent considered themselves vulnerable to contracting herpes, sixty-three percent indicated they were adopting precautions, and twenty-two percent said they had altered their sexual behavior to avoid the risk of contracting herpes. Only one percent of those contacted acknowledged having the disease, but eighty percent had heard of it, most within the last two years. And in a separate survey taken by the Herpes Resource Center, twenty-one percent of the herpes victims questioned said they had been rejected after confiding in prospective sexual partners. Lacking was information on those who chose not to reveal to their sex partners that they had contracted herpes.

This fact could be disquieting for those persons free of herpes who believe they are protected by vigilant observation of sexual partners for blisters; the disease is transferable, supposedly, only during an outbreak of these lesions. Unfortunately, there are victims who are capable of transferring herpes without having eternal symptoms or during the less obvious phase of viral shedding preceding an outbreak of blisters. Also, though helpful, the condom does not cover the entire genital area.

Two "herpes fraud" lawsuits have been filed by women who "trusted" their sex partners. The first was a married woman in North Carolina who sued her husband for $3 million on the grounds that he gave her herpes. It's not surprising that a married person would sue a mate after contracting an incurable venereal disease. Less expected was the $100,000 lawsuit filed in Florida by an unmarried woman who contracted herpes from a partner after she asked, "Am I going to catch anything from you?" As of this printing these two suits have yet to be settled. Would we all climb into our beds—or someone else's—feeling safer if these two were to win their lawsuits?

If you were poking around looking for a herpe, what would it look like? If you suspected you were harboring a herpe, what would it feel like? In *The Herpes Book*, Richard Hamilton, M.D., gives a graphic description worth remembering:

> The first sign of herpes that most people notice is a tingling, itching, or burning sensation near the site of the developed infection. The surface appears slightly discolored and is almost invariably sensitive to touch. Within hours . . . occasionally a day or two may pass, one or more small red marks will appear on the affected surface. These marks will resemble a measles rash, but they are confined to a very small area. . . . In a very short time . . . the small red marks develop into fluid-

filled, blisterlike sores that appear watery and grayish at the center and red around the edges. The entire area near the sores may be swollen and inflamed, and the pain may be quite sharp, radiating outward to adjacent areas . . . [many experience] swollen lymph glands, muscle aches, malaise, and fever. Over the next two to ten days the fluid-filled sores will gradually perforate and begin to "weep." Before a scab forms, the weeping sore may appear to be punched-out or ulcerlike. . . . As new mucus membrane or skin develops, the scabs fall off and, generally, by the end of the second week most patients are almost completely recovered—or so it may appear.

Hamilton's last phrase gives us the "herpes hitch." It's one thing to have a case of genital herpes once in your life. It's something else again when the scarlet pimple returns and stabs you over and over and over again—sometimes up to five or six times a year for years to come. The good news is, for those fifty percent who suffer from recurrent attacks, the first attack is the longest and the meanest. After that, lesions hang around about five days and viral shedding tacks on another five. The bad news is: some victims are sexually inactive up to sixty days a year—*if* they care enough to protect their sex partner from sharing their fate. Add to this the psychological trauma experienced by most herpes victims who suffer from recurrent attacks. In a survey of 7,500 patients, the American Social Health Association found that thirty-five percent experienced impotence or diminished sex drive.

Of all twenty-some venereal diseases that get under our skin, Puritans have chosen genital herpes as the STD that nature (God?) has chosen to halt "an era of mindless promiscuity." And some claim the media must be in cahoots with them because of their massive coverage of a tiny cold sore.

Still one would imagine Mother Nature—or someone even more influential—would threaten "mindless promiscuity" with a weightier weapon than a recurring scarlet pimple, or the shame of having one (sorry, the shame of sex still sticks, because the theory that genital herpes can be contracted from towels and toilets appears to be going down the drain). As for the media adopting a puritanical attitude about promiscuity, one has only to view any prime-time TV series to realize that media interests lie in getting males cockeyed with their sex objects and they are not cocking around with the vagaries of a scarlet pimple to cure a "mindless" popular indoor (usually) sport.

One thing about promiscuity—it takes up little of a person's leisure time, or so a recent survey indicates. Copulation was seventeenth on a list of how Americans spent their off hours. It came right after gardening.

Another threat, far more deadly, has surfaced in the last few years. It's a virus that produces AIDS—Acquired Immune Deficiency Syndrome—and it zeroed in primarily on the male homosexual community. AIDS destroys the immune systems geared to protect the human body from infectious diseases. The disease was first diagnosed in New York City in 1980 and no one thought a lot about it, since the first victims were Haitian aliens. However, by early 1983 the situation had drastically changed. The male gay communities in New York and San Francisco were spreading the word that lovers and friends were dying of an incurable disease. Actually, they were the victims of fatal diseases such as Kaposi's sarcoma, a rare form of cancer, and PCP (*Pneumocystis carinii* pneumonia), a rare respiratory infection that became associated with AIDS.

And, the gay community had good reason for their frantic concern since medical statistics eventually showed that seventy-two percent of AIDS victims were male homosexuals. The other twenty-eight percent were divided between intravenous drug users; people who had received blood transfusions from an AIDS victim; and Haitian immigrants to the United States.

After further research it was discovered that sperm entering the anal canal could be absorbed into a person's lymphatic and blood circulation systems, where they *may* set up an immune response as if they were invading infectious agents. From the time of this "discovery" AIDS was put on the list for sexually transmitted diseases. It is also spread by other bodily fluids, i.e., blood.

Sex or no sex, AIDS has an alarming fatality rate and no cure is in sight (despite a discovery in April 1984 of an AIDS-related virus—HTLV-III).

In mid-November of 1984 the Centers for Disease Control in Atlanta reported the total number of AIDS cases nationwide was 6,993, and that throughout 1984, the number of AIDS cases reported had increased seventy-four percent compared to the same period of 1983. Add to that the grim statistic that the death toll has increased along with the number of cases. In 1983 the fatality rate was forty-one percent. In 1984 this rate increased to forty-eight percent. In less than two years' time 3,342 persons have died from this dread disease.

10

THE PENILE COLONY

"The Love that dare not speak its name" in this century is such a great affection of an elder man for a younger man as there was between David and Jonathan, such as Plato made the basis of his philosophy and such as you find in the sonnets of Michelangelo and Shakespeare. It is that deep spiritual affection that is as pure as it is perfect. . . . There is nothing unnatural about it.

—Oscar Wilde, 1895

"What most people don't understand is that there is no such thing as *the* homosexual, that homosexual men and women can be as different as heterosexuals are from each other" (Alan P. Bell, psychologist, Institute for Sex Research, Indiana University, Bloomington, September 1978).

131

"The word *homosexual* is a rather meaningless word as a social concept. It cannot tell us how, under what conditions, when, or why a homosexual acts; nor does the word specify a type of person. . . . Social customs, norms, and the rules governing homosexual behavior are as varied as the number of persons engaged in such behavior" (James W. Chesebro, *GAYSPEAK*, 1981).

The above three quotations, nearly a century apart, tell us how far we've come—from a two-year jail sentence—and how far we still have to go—acceptance of the homosexual as one of "us" (humans who eat, shit, love, and—with any luck—fuck till the day we die).

Homosexual activity outside of the human race—which some scientists prefer calling "inversion"—few give a damn about. A majority of urban-bred humans can't distinguish between the sexes in animals other than dogs and cats. Also, it takes a bit of skilled eyeballing to spot the gender in those species where homosexual activity runs "rampant"—bedbugs, geese, Belgian carrier pigeons, and a bug who pops up under the scientific name of *Xylocaris maculipennis*.

Only those blessed with an open mind should take up in-depth bird-watching since birdland abounds with homosexual activity. So prevalent is it that man's earliest symbol for homosexuality is Egyptian—the symbol of two male partridges doing it.

Three thousand centuries have passed since the origin of this early symbol, and man has amassed a packet of terminology to describe the homosexual and his sexual activities. Most of these come under the category of vicious name-calling by evil-disposed heterosexuals. But some, equally brutal, originate from homosexuals themselves.

Here are gathered together some of these terms and euphemisms—both friendly and hostile—used to describe the homosexual and homosexual activity.

Those who have an aversion to name-calling are advised to flip past the next few pages.

132

SYNONYMS AND EUPHEMISMS FOR HOMOSEXUALITY

VICE SQUAD

Gross indecency
Abominable offenses
Nameless acts
Indecent assault
Unspeakable crimes
Abnormality
Unmentionable vice
Unnatural connection
Unnatural purposes
Unnatural vice
Unnatural offense
Unnatural sexual intercourse
An unmentionable crime
   against man and beast
Hollywood and Greenwich
   Village sodomists
Crime against nature
Unnatural debauchee
Odious vice
Unchaste
Nameless crime

HINDSIGHTING

Bung-holing
A bit of brown
Boody
Wages of a dog
Brown hatters
Stern-chaser

HINDSIGHTING (*cont'd.*)

Backscuttle
Fart-catcher
Butt-fuck
Shit-stir
The act of a beast

HEADHUNTERS

Chicken cannibal
Dirty old man
Third sexer
Sheepherder
Active sodomist
Shit-hunter

PSYCHOLOGICAL WARFARE

Higher Malthusianism
Sexual anomaly
Sexual perversion
Inversion
Perversion
Polymorphous perverse
Psychic hermaphrodite

NATIONAL HIT LIST

Greek love
Prussian love
Spanish love
Turk
English-style
Love in Italy

NATIONAL HIT LIST (*cont'd.*)
The Polish way
Persians
Syrians

BELLE OF THE BALLS
Angelina
Fairy Fay
Nellie
Sweetie
Dolly
Betty
Foxy lady
Pussy Nell
Nola
Mary
Ethel
Daisy
Nancy
Rimadonna
Belle

SAFE HOUSE
The closet
A renter
Enter the back door
Gentlemen of the back door
Back-door work
Bunker
Lick box
Gear box

BOYS IN THE BAND
Charlie
Joey
Willie
Skippy
Oscar
Flute
Orchestra

PINCH HITTERS
Oddball
Four-letter man
Joy boy
Jocker
Man's man
Fancy man
Peter pansy
Three-letter man
Fly ball
Gay boy
One of those

A SLICE OF LIFE
Gay
Funny
Ginger beer
Tickle your fancy
Backgammon
Daub of the brush
A bit of navy cake

A SLICE OF LIFE (cont'd.)

Dip in the fudge pot
Glory hole
Buggah
Gentlemen's games
Gaycat
Brighton Pier
Leather
Cowboy
Homoerotic
Cruising
Ship's shit-fuck

BIG SHOTS

Arse king
Queen
Drag queen
Brownie king
Mason
The endorser

MOLES

Bug
Wolf
Fugitive from a daisy-chain
    gang
Brown eye-brown hole
Undercover man
Muzzle
Q.
Insertee
Inspector

MOLES (cont'd.)

The Buzzer
K.
Closet queen
Closet queer
Antsypay
Buggery

DOUBLE AGENTS

He/she
Him/her
AC/DC
Twank/Twink
Green and yellow fellow

DEAR ONES

Sister
Daddy
Auntie
Uncle
Daughter
Mother
Baby

A ZOO

Bird taker
Three-legged beaver
Meat hound
Mouser
Bird

A ZOO (cont'd.)
Fruit fly
Birdie
Bait
Bestiality
Bugger
Capon

BODY LANGUAGE

Homogenitalism
Ass-fuck
Fist-fuck
Kisser
Light-footed
Gut-vexer
Light on his feet
Man-made woman
Uranus
Broken-wrist
Limp-wrist
Gut-stretcher
Gut-stuffer
Eye doctor
Eye opener
Gut-fucker
Back-hole
Ambidextrous
Gut-monger
To defile the mouth
A wasting spiritual disease
Buyer of masculine flesh
Bent

EATING OUT

Brownie
Quince
Fruitcake
Fruitplate
Chicken
Fruit
In the biscuit
Hairburger
Gooser
Hock
Bun
Fruiter
Corn-holer
Stuffer

A BOUQUET

Buttercup
Flower
Lily
Pansy

CONSUMER GOODS

Bag
Gobbler
Bottle
Basket

SCORCHING

Bitch
Freak
Fag
Faggot
Faggart
Kweer
Sissy
Mo
Pederast
Swish
Dinge
Thing
Pig-sticking
Ram-job
Cocksucking faggot
Bum fucker
Lewd

SCARY

Odd
Oddball
Screaming fairy
Weird
Badling
Keister stab
A fundamental debilitating
   factor in any civilization
Alien sex

GONIFS

Bandit
Crimes
Burglar
Con
Punk
Shim
Midnight cowboy
Night sneakers
Ring snatcher
Three-dollar bill

GOBBLEDYGOOK

Agfay
Pood
Secko
Spurge
Eer-quay
Fluter
Jere
Larro
Mintie
Pads
Dyna
Punce
Poofter
Aspro
Fooper
Frit
Gonsel
Farg
Dinge

GOBBLEDYGOOK (*cont'd.*)

Quadean
Quean
Wonk
Afgay
Pedication
Anarieis
Stuprum
Inglar
Bud sallogh
Vert
Padeagogia
Cinaedus
Paedicator
Paiderasty
Cadamite
Pathiksos
Pathics
Couus
Masculorum concubitores
Slupurm
Coitus in ano
Coitus per anum
Crimen innomminatum
Concubitis cum persona
  ejudsen sexus
Paedicatio
Hat hesh
Urningin
Urning
Sod

RELIGIOUS/BIBLICAL

Sodomist
Sodomite

RELIGIOUS/BIBLICAL (*cont'd.*)

Jesuit
Wages of a dog
Defile themselves with
  mankind
Monstrous and unnatural
  vices of hededom
Sin against nature
Kneeling at the altar

GOOD NEWS

Come out
Bring out
The Greek way
Corvette
Inspirer
The beloved
The listener
The wooer
To educate
Ideal love
The passive role/the active
  role
The sphere of the beautiful
True boy love
Cut sleave

AND THE BAD NEWS

To outrage
To dishonor
To carry out infamous
  conduct
To be full of impurity

AND THE BAD NEWS (*cont'd.*)

To have despicable habits
Curse of the feminine disease
Defilement
Violation
One who submits to
  unnatural lust
Step-child of nature
Subactor
Subjugate
To work
The things that are done by
  them in secret, it is a
  shame even to speak of
Vile affection
Abusers of themselves
Unlawful mixture
Unpardonable insult to
  nature

IMAGE CONSULTANTS

Jockey
Chi-chi
Dandy
Femme
Girl
Other sex
Truck driver
Himmer
Spintry
Bucklebury
Nancie-homie
Horse's hoof
Sweet

IMAGE CONSULTANTS (*cont'd.*)

Puff
Usher
Size queen
Clone
Inspector of man holes

HEAVENLY BODIES

Angel
Pixie
Mince
Trick
Flutter

NIELSEN RATING

Boys
Gay-boy
Jocker
Effeminate male
Pervert
Kinky
That way
Queer
Queervert
Homo
Homie
Homophile

FRINGE BENEFITS

Lacy
Pure silk
Lavender

FRINGE BENEFITS (*cont'd.*)
Lay
Ship's sodomy
Nigh enough
Pouffe
Camp
Lavender boy

???
Homosexual
Sexual orientation
Sexual preference
Gay

COUNTERINTELLIGENCE

Not interested in the
  opposite sex

Despite the stretch—and the stench—of this lengthy list, homosexuals, always a minority, lived side by side with heterosexuals for centuries without having a label slapped on them. And the reason for this is basic. Prehistoric man was not blind. Homosexual activity occurs in most species of herd animals when the male is separated from the female. With both feet on the ground, prehistoric man rationalized, these animals had it pegged just right.

Early man was isolated from the female for lengthy periods during his hard-fought existence. Hunting, exploring, fighting wars, transporting food and materials were tasks that took ages to complete when all had to be done by putting one foot in front of another. Having women along was seldom practical. Man turned to man for sex and personal contact, uninhibited by the taboos of religion or moralists.

Evidence of homosexuality goes as far back as prehistoric cave paintings and as late as 3100 B.C. in the tombs of ancient Egypt, a broad hint that some of these pharaohs enjoyed homosexual activity so much that they intended to still be doing it in the next life.

The first known language symbol for homosexual activity comes from ancient Greece: *paiderastes*, later anglicized as pederasty, which derives from the Greek terms for *boy* and *lover.* Havelock Ellis says this term was made honorable around 1100 B.C. by the Dorians, invaders from northern Greece who overran the entire Greek peninsula and Asia Minor. Among unsparing Spartans, *paiderastia* meant the hookup of a young male between the age of twelve and sixteen with an experienced warrior who yearned to teach the uninitiated lad about life with a capital *L* and battle. In benevolent Crete, *paiderastia* involved introducing a willing lad to an idyllic honeymoon on which he first would be wined and dined in a romantic setting for weeks before learning about courage and valor on the battlefield.

Ancient Greeks, like many of their gods, favored a bisexual existence. The ideal pattern for earthlings naturally had to be more practical. As a young lad, a fortunate boy experienced a homosexual affair (or two). As a young adult, he would turn to the heterosexual experience to propagate the race and round out his sexual sensations. As a mature adult, he was responsible for the training—sensual and pragmatic—of a youth worthy (not a slave, for God's sake!) of such a well-rounded education from such a well-rounded educator.

But these gay escapades of the Greeks were a shade less honorable in the eyes of their Roman conquerors. The Romans began making a hefty list of not so nice (or polite) names to tag homosexual activity and homosexuals. *Struprum* was a term that stood for both homosexual and heterosexual "improper" sexual intercourse. But *cinaedi* singled out the homosexual as "unmanly." *Catamiti* (anglicized today, *catamite* means a boy kept for "unnatural purposes") stood for passive male homosexuals and *exoleti* (accelerant?) stood for active male prostitutes.

Ancient Greece had class. It was a culture dedicated to a quest for truth, from the vast expanse of the universe to the intimate and the sexual. But their Roman conquerors were out for power and powerful images. This macho perspective was used to negate the Greek influence in the West and Asia Minor. And one ax they used for severing this influence was promoting male Greeks as a bunch of pansies.

Bad-mouthing homosexual activity became a popular indoor sport, *almost* as popular as bisexual intercourse among the ruling classes. Historically, Julius Caesar was the first ruler of a powerful empire to be subjected to abusive ridicule for his AC/DC predilections. Romans openly chided the first Caesar for being "a husband of all women and a wife of all men."

But Caesars—twelve in all—were famous for never tuning into the chatter of the populace. In response to Edward Gibbon's statement in *The Decline and Fall of the Roman Empire* that "of the first fifteen emperors Claudius was the only one whose tastes in love was entirely correct" (meaning, of course, heterosexual), John Boswell, in *Christianity, Social Tolerance and Homosexuality*, gives us a healthy chuckle when he observes:

> If Gibbon was right, the Roman Empire was ruled for almost 200 consecutive years by men whose homosexual interests, if not exclusive, were sufficiently noteworthy to be recorded for posterity.

The Roman Empire crumpled and died in 476 A.D. Before its death, the vile labels slapped by Romans on homosexuals and homosexual activity had spread like a cancer through the West. But one vile label came from the once-classy Greeks.

In the second century A.D. a famed Greek physician, Soranus, labeled homosexual effeminate men as unnatural, diseased human beings. Caelius Aurelianus, a Latin translator, gives us this glimpse of Soranus's bludgeoning diagnoses of the victims, called *pathics.*

142

> People find it hard to believe that effeminate men or pathics (Greek *malthacoe*) really exist. The fact is that, though the practices of such persons are unnatural to human beings, lust overcomes modesty and puts to shameful use parts intended for other functions . . . there is no limit to their desire and no hope of satisfying it; and they cannot be content with their own lot. . . . They even adopt the dress, walk, and other characteristics of women. Now, this condition is different from a bodily disease; it is rather an affliction of a diseased mind. . . . For as Soranus says, this affliction comes from a corrupt and diseased mind.

Let us hope Soranus met some of these pathetic *pathics* in a dark alley some night. Somehow it doesn't seem fair that the first "sickie" label for homosexuals should come from a Greek who had no class.

And in the sixth century A.D. homosexuals suffered another first, Boswell tells us: until the sixth century, homosexual acts not covered by specific laws (i.e., statutory rape of minors and gay marriages) were legal, but then the Romans decided that that was not severe enough so they made *all* homosexual intercourse illegal.

As the world switched from B.C. to A.D., China had a healthier outlook. It was during this time the label "cut sleeve" became an endearing term for homosexual activity.

Ai Ti (6 B.C.–2 A.D.), one of the last Han emperors, a well-known "wooer" of lads, took a sword and cut the sleeve from his gown so as not to disturb his boy lover sleeping beside him, his head resting upon it. A class act, right?

But not in the evil eyes of many in the West, who began to tag homosexual intercourse as "the disease from the East." In fact the real disease was in the Western world, where homophobia began to spread like a plague from the paranoia of Jewish and early Christian prejudice against the Greek influence.

Idolatry and the Greek concept of life and how to live it were now considered evil and wicked. Even the Greeks were beginning to turn on their ancestral heritage. A tragic example of the switch from homosexual activity as an art to an act against nature lies in the origin of the mudslinging term sodomy.

Sodom was flattened in 1900 B.C. Modern historians claim the ancient city, along with Gomorrah and three other cities, was destroyed in a devastating earthquake that tore up most of the area south of the Dead Sea. Biblical commentators as early—actually late—as 105 B.C. claim Sodom got it because the city was populated with sex fiends. But the ancient original text of Deuteronomy, where the tale of these toppled cities first appears, never says a word about sex and devastation. So who slapped the original tag of sodomy on homosexual intercourse?

Appropriately, a man named Philo Judaeus, a Hellenic Egyptian Jew, in the first century A.D. Here's his description of the studs who populated Sodom (apparently only God knows what the studs in Gomorrah were up to):

> . . . applied themselves to . . . forbidden forms of intercourse. Not only in their mad lust for women did they violate the marriage of their neighbors, but also men mounted males without respect for sex nature which the active partner shares with the passive; so when they tried to beget children they were discovered to be incapable of any but a sterile seed. . . . Then little by little they accustomed those who were by nature men to submit to play the part of women. . . . For not only did they emasculate their bodies by luxury . . . they worked a further degeneration in their souls . . . corrupting the whole of mankind.

Well, that showed you where Judaeus was at—just about where the early Christians were. Sperm was for making babies, and those babies had better be conceived by your spouse or else you were a corrupting louse eating away at all of humanity.

In the twelfth century the Christian Church was faced with its first real threat. Heretics were popping up all over Europe. To combat the growing rebellion against Christian supremacy the church-controlled states of Europe resorted to the death penalty for those condemned as heretics.

By the thirteenth century, heresy in Italy and France was defined as the practice of devil worship, adultery, incest, or sodomy. A torturous example is the charge of sodomy and devil worship brought against the Knights Templar.

The Knights Templar originated in the twelfth century when eight French knights consecrated their lives to the protection of pilgrims as they toured the holy sites in Jerusalem. Muslim bands of robbers and murderers had made the trip to the Holy Land a holy terror for Christians. The eight knights gained the protection of the King of Jerusalem, who quartered the Christian knights in a Jewish temple (thus Templars). Tales of the knights' heroic deeds spread throughout the Christian world. When other knights joined their brave battle a decision was made to organize a religious military force of militant monks. Besides protecting the pilgrims, the Templars went into the banking biz as a method of money exchange and protection for the hassled tourist—a bit like American Express.

Protecting someone's money is a sure road to riches. In less than a century, the Templars had become a powerhouse. They continued their escort service but now more as a courtesy—and P.R.—since most of their time was taken up running a powerful army, buying real estate, and banking—giving loans with lower interest rates than other sharks. Their interest rates were so reasonable that governments began seeking out the Templars. Not bad for a bunch of noble knights who took the vow of poverty and chastity. But government loans wound up to be the undoing of the Templars.

By the beginning of the fourteenth century, the Knights were back in France doing their wheeling and dealing. They foolishly made loans to their avaricious king, Philip the Fair, taking no heed when the Fair one in 1306 expelled all the Jews from France, then proceeded to seize their property and all the bucks owed them.

In 1307 the Fair one, in debt to his socks with the Templars, issued an order to put every Knight in the royal jail. What was his charge? That the Knights indulged in homosexual lusts, spat on the cross as a sign of allegiance, and carried on sacrilegious rites where initiates had to kiss the ass of their sponsors and submit to passive copulation if a fellow Knight requested it.

Naturally, the Knights denied the charges. And naturally, the Fair one tortured them until most of the Knights confessed. Those who did not died or committed suicide after being hung by their wrists while their feet were roasted in flames, their teeth extracted one by one, splinters were driven under their fingernails, and being subjected to the ball breaker—weights hung from their genitals.

After three years of prison and torture, fifty-nine Knights were burned at the stake, including their leader Jacques de Molay, the Grand Master, who retracted his confession (as did others) while being led to his fiery death. And, fair as always, the king seized their estates and called in all their loans with the exception of his own.

One historian of the Inquisition called this "the crime of the century." Certainly, as a group, these knights were the first martyrs to die for homosexual activities—whether they did it or not.

For the next two centuries France had a persecution complex.

When the Black Death hit in the mid-fourteenth century the French persecuted friars and those brave Jews who returned to France after the death of the Fair one. But then everyone becomes edgy during difficult times, especially if their gods and religion fail to find a solution. The Church couldn't stop the plague, but it could come up with a scapegoat for frightened Frenchmen. This solution was par for the ecclesiastic course—give the poor bewildered souls something to *really* worry about. Witches, demons, and satanists provided the devilish solution. All of France went on a Halloween binge.

In 1431 Frenchmen cheered when their heroic savior, Joan of Arc, was burned at the stake for heresy and demonic practices. For not playing-it-all-girl, there were five separate charges relating to her preference for wearing male attire, both in and out of battle.

And nine years after Joan's death, one of her compatriots and protectors became the next possible martyr to French homophobia during the Middle Ages. We say possible, because to this day historians can't agree if Gilles de Rais was guilty or innocent of the charges made against him by the Church-controlled state.

Gilles de Rais was a Frenchman and a half. During his forty years he was a war hero, an aristocrat, an heir to millions in real estate and francs, Grand Marshall of France, patron of the arts, head honcho of a court so classy it turned the complexion of his poor French king green, a lifesaver (twice) and a guiding light for Joan of Arc in her battles to save the throne of Charles VII. He was also a mass murderer, a devil worshiper, and last, but far from least, a sodomist with a chilling preference for dead little boys.

The final three items on the above résumé are suspect to this day since they were among charges of heresy, etc., made by acquisitive inquisitors. According to the ecclesiastics, Gilles turned to satanism when his family succeeded in placing funds from his estates under government protection, claiming they were headed for bankruptcy because of his splendacious court. It was then, supposedly, that Gilles—proud as Lucifer—resorted to making human sacrifices to the devil in hopes of regaining control of his inheritance. These human sacrifices were all young boys who Gilles was accused of sexually molesting before and after their murders. How many lads? Since millions of francs were at stake, the murderous total came to somewhere between one hundred forty and two hundred innocent lads.

Arrested in 1440, Gilles was brought before both an ecclesiastic tribunal and a civil court. When he refused to confess to their charges, Gilles was threatened with excommunication and torture. Scholars now suspect that Gilles, recalling Joan's fiery death nine years earlier, tossed aside heroics and confessed, throwing himself on the mercy of the court. Mercifully, the ecclesiastics acclaimed Gilles a true Christian, for he had repented and was resigned to his own death by hanging.

It took the French another 370 years to get their sexual revolution together. In 1810 the Napoleonic Code was passed in France. The Code abolished all civil punishment for any sexual behavior between consenting adults, whether between man and woman, woman and woman, or man and man. Only those who ignored public decency or resorted to violence were hauled before a judge. This Code became law in most of Europe, since Napoleon was calling the shots on most of the Continent.

The British, Napoleon's conquerors, naturally turned their nose up at the mere thought of adapting their laws to anything that carried the whiff of their hated rival and opponent. Therefore, it comes as no surprise that an Englishman was the next famous martyr to be called a sodomist.

In 1895 the Marquess of Queensberry (don't let this title confuse you; he was so straight that he laid down the rules for boxing) sent a card to a famous London club addressed "To Oscar Wilde, Posing as a Somdomite." Despite the misspelling, Wilde recognized the insult and, in a sizzling rage, sued the Marquess for criminal libel. Three trials later Wilde was found guilty of several acts of gross indecency. The acts of gross indecency were perpetrated on, among others, one Lord Alfred Douglas, one of four male heirs to the Queensberry chattels.

Wilde's defense, in part, was the eloquent, moving statement quoted at the beginning of this chapter. It got him, as a convicted sodomist, two years of hard labor, exile in shame, and an early death.

Though the mores of Victorian England seem archaic to us, the echo of sodomy still rings out, since "sodomy laws" exist to this day in many American states. And, less than ten years ago, three states still carried a maximum penalty of life imprisonment for partaking of the "love that dare not speak its name."

The late nineteenth and twentieth centuries brought the scientific terms for homosexual activity and homosexuals. Most of these labels, no matter how well meaning, make homosexuals sound like escapees from a loony bin.

In 1875 Karl Heinrichs Ulrichs, a homosexual, came up with *urning* in honor of the Greek god Uranus, who sired the goddess of love. At the turn of the century the physician Carl Westphal became famous for his theories on "contrary sexual feeling." Then most of the medical profession began fooling around with the term *perversion*. Havelock Ellis, objecting to perversion, thought "sexual inversion" was more factual. Krafft-Ebing, never at a loss for words, favored "hereditary taint" and "moral degenerate" and all of the above. Researcher Edward Stevenson was caught up with "the intersexes" and "similisexualism," but then his middle name was Irenaeus. Magnus Hirshfield, a homosexual and the founder of the Institute for Sexual Science, coined *zwischen*, which translates into "intermediate state." And someone came up with "inverted sexual instinct."

Add to those this medicinal dose: "psychic hermaphrodite," "polymorphous perverse," "sexual anomaly," "higher Malthusianism," "homogenic love," "homo-eroticism," "sexual orientation," and "sexual preference."

The word *homosexual* originated in the late nineteenth century but only came into popular use decades later. It was coined by a German psychologist as a humane definition for any male who preferred having sex with another male. Today most gays consider the term simplistic, confusing, and, above all, negative.

The term *gay* has a complex origin dating as far back as the thirteenth century and the days of courtly love. Troubadour poetry and songs were both written and popularized by homosexuals in the south of France and persisted through the centuries as a slang term for "the gay life," which in some regions included female prostitutes. Somewhere in the 1950s "gay" became the preferred term among persons "who are conscious of an erotic preference for their own sex."

Whatever the term chosen, finally, gays are telling the world who, what, and where they are. *And* what to call them.

So why, might you be asking, was the term *homosexual* used throughout this choky chapter on the etymological history of homosexuality? Because *gay* is the one term that doesn't stick in your throat, and we all like a happy ending.

11

THE ADVENTURE OF THE ODD BALL AND OTHER BONES OF CONTENTION

Hitler has only got one ball,
Göring has two but very small,
Himmler has something
  similar,
But poor Goebbels has no balls
  at all.
    —Brendan Behan, Borstal Boy

And then there are the ballsy male genitals that become legends in their own time. And even more ballsy are those that refuse with the passage of time to drop by the wayside.

Brendan Behan's ditty, quoted above, was sung by boys in a reform school in the early 1940s. With the exception of Behan, no one, including historians, gave a twitch about Hitler's balls until a quarter of a century later. In May 1968, almost twenty-three years to the day after Hitler's death, the USSR released the autopsy report for the German Führer and his wife, Eva Braun Hitler.

Now there are those prejudiced against anything Red who claim that all Russians are slow-witted and have the IQ of a cat. Others, more magnanimous, scratched their heads and wondered if by chance this might be a diabolic plot to prove Hitler did not die after all in his Berlin bunker. And others—historians, physicians, and intimate friends of the dictator—*knew* foul play was afoot, after studying the much belated report.

What, in this autopsy report, sparked once again the fantasy that the Führer had survived the war? One was an outrageous claim that Hitler's body, though noticeably damaged by fire, had no visible signs of a lethal injury or severe illnesses and that he died, as did Eva, from cyanide compounds in a crushed glass ampule found in the oral cavity. Period. This claim was made despite the documented eyewitness accounts of those Germans who later testified Hitler died from a bullet in his head.

But, since the report admits a piece of the cranium was missing, there were those who pooh-poohed the Russian "interpretation" of the method used by Hitler for suicide.

What really opened a can of worms was the report that Hitler was minus his left testicle (yes, one does hang portside while the other dangles starboard). The forensic scientists said they searched, to no avail, for the missing testicle in the scrotum, the spermatic cord inside the inguinal canal, and the small pelvis.

Now, Hitler's physicians, intimate friends, and lovers were all willing—after the war—to call Hitler an oddball upstairs. But downstairs he was a normal male. The Führer had one penis, two testicles, and he enjoyed the usual exercise—sexual—that kept everything in good shape. A hole in the head from a bullet could be overlooked with a damaged cranium, but a missing testicle! Forget it! You don't misplace those things and you never lose count of them!

152

And suddenly the worm turned. If not the Führer's, whose body was it? And, even more important, where was Hitler's? Did he escape the bunker? Was he still alive?

The question of the missing testicle resurrected questions about Hitler's death.

For those who couldn't give a swat how the old blabbermouth got it or care if he lost a nut along the way, the next page or two will seem tedious; others might enjoy testing their analytical talents.

On May 1, 1945, Joseph Goebbels sent a telegram from the Führer-bunker to Admiral Karl Dönitz announcing Dönitz was the new German head of state because Hitler had ended his life at 3:30 P.M. on April 30. On May 3 and 4 the Soviet Army retrieved four charred corpses from the ruins above the bunker. On June 6 the Russians announced that one of the corpses was the body of Adolf Hitler (the other three were presumed to be Eva Braun Hitler, and Joseph and Magda Goebbels). On June 9 in Berlin the Russians announced at a press conference, "We did not identify the body of Hitler. I [Marshal Zhukov] can say nothing definite about his fate. He could have flown away from Berlin at the very last moment. The state of the runway would allow him to do so."

Zhukov also announced that they were unable to find the body of Martin Bormann, Hitler's personal secretary and head of the Nazi Party, who had been in the bunker with his leader until the final day.

In July, General Dwight Eisenhower was quoted replying to the question "Are you convinced Hitler's dead?" "To tell the truth, I'm not. I was at first . . . But when I actually got to talk to my Russian friends, I found they weren't convinced."

In August 1945 at the Potsdam Conference, Stalin, after a request to state his views on how Hitler died, told President Harry Truman and Secretary of State James Byrnes, "I believe Hitler is alive. Careful research by Soviet investigators has not found any trace of Hitler's remains or any positive evidence of his death." Stalin went on to say he believed Hitler should be listed as a war criminal and sentenced to death by hanging.

Since there was no *corpus delicti*, British and U.S. governments could only nod in agreement when the Russians blabbed to the world that Hitler must be alive and in hiding. The Führerbunker had been captured by the Soviets and it remained after the war strategically in the Russian zone of Berlin.

In the fall of 1945 the Soviets accused the Brits of hiding Hitler and Eva Braun in the British zone. With that kick in the teeth, the British, with the Yanks in tow, decided to investigate for themselves how, or if, Hitler escaped death in the bunker. The sleuth employed by the British was one Hugh Trevor-Roper. (In 1983, he authenticated the forged diaries of Hitler, but whistled another tune when handwriting experts proved the diaries were as queer as a $7 bill.) Trevor-Roper, with the assist of Michael Musmanno for the U.S., interviewed the survivors of the Führerbunker who had escaped being captured by the Soviets. The conclusion of the investigators was that: Hitler was as dead as a doornail and he died on April 30, 1945, in a suicide pact with his bride Eva Braun Hitler. He pumped a bullet in his head and she chomped a cyanide capsule. Following Hitler's command, their bodies were burned in the garden above the bunker. The following day, Joseph and Magda Goebbels did a suicide duet after poisoning their six children, and Martin Bormann was killed while attempting to flee from the Russian forces.

Trevor-Roper produced a nice neat package. But, other than the British government, no one gave a hoot. There was still the problem of no *corpus delicti*. No one, including the government, questioned the fact that Trevor-Roper made his report without even visiting the burial site in his brief seven weeks of sleuthing.

So rumors continued to fly around the world that the

Satan of the twentieth century was still alive. Magazines and newspapers reported Hitler and Eva were alive and well in Japan, Argentina, the Vatican, the palace of an Arab sheikh, etc. etc. etc. Even the *Encyclopaedia Britannica* and *The New York Times Index* played it cool, listing Hitler as b. 1889, d. 1945?

And then the Soviets in 1968 released their oddball autopsy report. And to confuse things even more, they had the chutzpah to admit that after poking around with Hitler's remains, they cremated his body in 1947 and threw his ashes to the winds.

Still no *corpus delicti!* And even if there had been one, it was missing a ball!

It's no wonder that to this day—forty years later and, for the nonce, minus a corpse—the world still remains in doubt about how, and when—not to mention if—Hitler died. In 1984 most people believe Hitler is decidedly dead or tottering on his graveside. At ninety-five Hitler is no longer a threat—at least not personally. But the world loves a mystery *and* a solution. So books are still being written, and read, describing the final solution for Hitler and Eva Braun.

Perhaps the real mystery is why the Russians released an autopsy report saying Hitler had only one ball. Maybe they believed Behan's trashy ditty, widely known since the 1958 publication of *Borstal Boy* and sung in many a pub to the tune of "The Bridge on the River Kwai."

Rasputin was born seventeen years before Hitler. And he died at the age of forty-four, while Hitler, at the age of twenty-seven, was serving as a lowly corporal in the German army during World War I. Hitler's penis was half the length of Rasputin's. There's a definite probability that if their measurements had been reversed, the twentieth century could have gone down in history as the golden age of progress rather than slaughter.

In 1906 the infant heir to the throne of Russia was

slowly bleeding to death while court physicians clucked that the babe, a hemophiliac, was not long for this world. Desperate, the infant's parents, the tsar and tsarina, appealed to a monk who had gained an awesome reputation as a faith healer—*and* a Casanova *and* a boozer *and* a clairvoyant *and* a living saint *and* a devil with a hell of a horn *and* a fornicator *and* a hypnotist *and* a rapist *and* a scummy peasant with BO *and*—as his delirious wife cried, he "has enough for all"—a thirteen-incher.

While a teenager this pushy buck was tagged "the seducer," which in Russian comes out Rasputin. The monicker is appropriate to the bone since Rasputin, besides being a seducer of women, was an *artiste* when it came to using hypnotic suggestion for seducing the mind.

René Fülöp-Miller, Rasputin's biographer, chronicles Rasputin's artistry in both of these areas when he quotes a young female disciple's first mind-blasting encounter with this horny monk:

> His gentle monastic gaze . . . at first inspired her with confidence. But when he came closer . . . she felt immediately that another quite different man, mysterious, crafty, and corrupting, looked out from behind the eyes that radiated goodness and gentleness. . . . A keen glance reached her from the corner of his eyes, bored into her, and held her fascinated. A sudden heaviness overpowered her limbs as his great wrinkled face, distorted with desire, came close to hers. She felt his hot breath on her cheeks, and saw how his eyes, burning from the depths of their sockets, furtively roved over her helpless body. . . . His voice had fallen to a passionate whisper. . . . Just as she was on the point of abandoning herself to her seducer . . . she recalled that she had come to ask him about God . . . she struggled . . .

Since this is not a romance novel, let's pull the plug before we all get overheated.

The problem with Rasputin, in addition to his meandering penis, was his erratic flip-flopping from a Jekyll to a Hyde. He rapes a nun, next day he falls in a saintly trance and cures the heir to the throne. One day he is dragging women into his "holy of holies" (his bed), the next he's lighting the tsarina's candles and leading prayers at the imperial altar.

The seduction of the imperial family was a natural for Rasputin. All he had to do was perform an eyewashing miracle—put Prince Aleksey in a hypnotic trance whenever he was in danger of bleeding to death.

Seduction of the imperial court was quite another thing. For one thing he smelled and perversely flaunted his gross peasant origins. Behind the backs of the tsar and tsarina, the court snickered that Rasputin was born in a barn, smelled the same, stank the court up with his barnyard expressions, and crowed like a cocky rooster as he recounted the numerous nobles he had put out to pasture as cuckolds.

To boot, Rasputin was at odds with the vast human ocean of Russian peasants. These peasants were just beginning to make their stand against imperial oppression. And there, in the midst of the hated court, batting the breeze with the despised nobles, was one of their own sticking out like the son of a sow. The peasants not only hated his guts, they hated his "gift." In a life devoid of sophistication *and* downright necessities, they reckoned a monk ought to act like a holy man instead of a barnyard stud. By 1914 the peasants had a new nickname for Rasputin—the Antichrist, the Man of Sin.

In his book *Dark Dimensions*, Welsh author Colin Wilson reveals that Rasputin was knifed in the gut by a peasant woman who screamed, "I have killed the Antichrist!" at the exact moment (2:15 P.M., July 28, 1914) that the heir to the Austrian throne, Archduke Ferdinand, and his wife were assassinated in Sarajevo. Those two shots rocketed the world into war.

Wilson claims that, of all the tsar's advisers, Rasputin

could have prevented Nicholas II's order for national mobilization, which precipitated Germany's declaration of war on Russia. Proof of Rasputin's influence over the tsar goes back to a time six years earlier when Rasputin prevented Russia from entering the Balkan War. The monk switched the tsar from a hawk to a dove with the single phrase, "The Balkans are not worth the life of a single Russian soldier."

When Rasputin regained consciousness from his near-fatal wound, he telegraphed a similar message to Nicholas. But, tragically, he spoke his peace too late.

Russia stayed in the war for three years, but Germany stayed till the bitter end. When Germany lost the war, its foundation rocked and crumbled, and this shockwave brought on the tidal wave of Nazi Germany.

And that's how one devious member's deviations can be blamed for getting a large portion of this globe into two world wars.

To Rasputin's credit, until his dying day, he was never a party pooper. Getting the horny monk to meet his maker reads like a final chapter from a James Bond thriller.

By 1916 Rasputin had enemies all over Russia. Even the monk sensed that his days were numbered. Proof lies in this letter he wrote to the tsarina, in which he predicted his own death. Unfortunately, his seer's power was too nearsighted to spot who the bugger was that would finally snuff him out.

> I feel I shall leave life before January 1. [Rasputin was murdered on December 29] . . . If I am killed . . . by my brothers the Russian peasants, you, tsar of Russia, have nothing to fear for your children, they will reign for hundreds of years in Russia. But if I am murdered by nobles . . . if it was your relations that wrought my death, then no one of your family . . . will remain alive for more than two years. They will be killed by the Russian people . . . I shall be killed. I am no longer among the living. [The tsar and his wife and five children were

assassinated by Bolshevik soldiers on July 18, 1918, nineteen and a half months after Rasputin's death.]

Now, guess who did Rasputin in. A bisexual husband of the tsar's niece. Yusupov, a prince of the empire, angered after Rasputin rebuffed his sexual advances, plotted with four other nobles—perhaps of more noble intention—to rid the Romanovs and Russia of the poisonous power of the horny monk.

Cunningly the prince invited Rasputin to meet his beautiful wife, the Princess Irina, the tsar's niece. Yusupov knew Rasputin couldn't resist the temptation of a possible new conquest. Rasputin arrived dressed to the nines in peasant apparel with a designer twist: a tunic of embroidered satin and velvet breeches. The prince, apologizing for his wife's delay, proceeded to serve Rasputin cakes and wines his co-conspirators had loaded with potassium cyanide.

Rasputin gobbled and gulped enough cyanide to put away a dozen men. Yet the monk, though fried to his eyes, remained fit while Yusupov fiddled. The prince, panicking when he realized Rasputin was impervious to the cyanide, belted off to his fellow assassins, who were on call to dispose of the monk's body, for advice. They handed him a pistol and told him to shoot.

According to Patte Barham, who collaborated on a biography of Rasputin with the monk's daughter, Maria, Yusupov pumped four bullets into the tiddly monk *after* raping him. The five assassins gathered around the stretched-out Rasputin in the mood for a fling; they castrated the monk and pitched his penis the length of the room.

The assassins then disposed of what they believed to be Rasputin's corpse under the ice of a frozen river. Discovered two days later, an autopsy proved Rasputin died, not from poison, not from bullets, not from brutal castration, not from the shock of being raped, but from drowning.

159

And what about his bigger-than-life thirteen-incher?

Last reported it was seen lying-in-state inside a polished wooden box (eighteen by six inches) on a bureau top in a lady's bedroom in Paris. It was fifty-two years after Rasputin's murder and how his thirteen-incher came to this appreciative haven is another story. More to the point, from this story's perspective, how was it holding up?

As one might suspect it was pooped. He was stretched out on a black piece of velvet. Still his same regal length but, here comes the downer, The Whopper now resembled, instead of a penis, a blackened, over-ripe banana.

Why did Napoleon's penis, once considered a better-than-average battering ram, end up resembling a fragment of grapeshot before the conqueror of most of Europe reached the age of fifty?

For close to thirty years Napoleon had twenty mistresses, countless one-night stands, and two wives (one considered just this side of a nympho). True, in the sack this world beater never gained the reputation of a sensual revolutionist, but he did have royal honors throughout the courts of Europe as the ruler who most enjoyed doing it. So why, at the age of forty-nine, do some historians claim Napoleon had met his sexual Waterloo? (Others claim Napoleon was impotent as early as the age of forty-two, but that has to be pushing it, for how else can one explain the late-night escapades of an adventurous adulteress who slid nightly for the better part of four years into Napoleon's bedroom on the island of Saint Helena?)

Albine de Montholon was in her mid-thirties when she accompanied her husband, Count Charles-Tristan de Montholon, to the remote island in the South Atlantic. Napoleon was sent into exile at the far-from-impotent age of forty-six.

Saint Helena was a ten-mile strip of nowheresville.

Why, if you weren't under the penalty of exile, would anyone opt for going there? The answer is, you had to be a manic-Napoleonic.

Surprisingly, after his blasting defeat, there were plenty of those manics clamoring to remain by their leader's side when he was sent into exile. But the British allowed the ex-emperor only five *male* companions, plus their wives and servants, to accompany him. Napoleon was very selective. He was posed with the problem some of us fantasize about: If you had to spend the rest of your life on a deserted isle, what would you take with you?

To protect his vanity, Napoleon chose his devoted valet. To protect his bod, a military officer who risked his life in Russia to save his emperor. To make sure his household ran smoothly, the one-time grand marshal of the Tuileries palace (who brought along a young, good-looking wife). To make sure history got a glimpse of his perspective, his own biographer, a scholarly count.

And last, but far from least, Count Montholon, a gentleman willing to share his sexy wife, Albine, who was also the willing kind. The count's wife suited Napoleon's needs to a T. The British would never suspect, until well after he was established on the island, that Napoleon had brought along a bed warmer. Another plus—the countess's sexual history closely mimicked that of his first wife, the sex-mad Josephine. With one difference: Josephine had been the mistress of several men before Napoleon married her. Albine, on the other hand, preferred to switch husbands; Montholon was her third. And, despite the generous leeway of the Napoleonic Code, three years previously Napoleon had banned Montholon from his imperial court for choosing this questionable lady as his bride. But, with exile and celibacy staring him in the eye, Albine Montholon was looking better and better to the former emperor.

And the cuckold count? Why was he so eager to join

Napoleon in exile? Until Napoleon's sentence to exile in Saint Helena, Montholon was never considered much more than a hanger-on in the imperial court. He was decidedly the type who hung around for the good times and their goodies. Saint Helena was a labor of mad love not up the count's alley at all.

Was Napoleon suspicious of Montholon's motives? Apparently not. So off Napoleon sailed to the drecky island with his British guardians and his five necessities. In a year the British shipped back the scholarly count, despite Napoleon's protests. Within three years, Napoleon's trusted bodyguard had left the island voluntarily, whining that he had no woman. Napoleon, the sneak, retorted, "Bah! Women! When you don't think about them, you don't need them. Be like me."

But his bodyguard, Gourgaud, had caught the accommodating Albine sneaking into Napoleon's bedroom. Albine would also blatantly join Napoleon while he lay soaking in his tub, shooing out his valet or her husband as they attended him. Albine was beginning to act like the Empress of Saint Helena.

Gourgaud considered Albine and her actions depraved. And the nonaction of her husband even more depraved. In his diary Gourgaud wrote before his departure, "Poor Montholon! What role are you playing?"

Indeed what was his role? A recent book, *The Murder of Napoleon*, tells a fantastic tale, but relays a more than probable solution to the mystery of Count Montholon's presence on Saint Helena. Montholon was sent to the island to slowly poison Napoleon.

Napoleon's health was gradually deteriorating. His British guardians thought he was faking at first. But symptoms surfaced which could not be faked. Swelling of his legs and ankles, vomiting, a persistent dry cough, a progressive gain in weight despite acute pains in the stomach, a yellow cast to his skin, and so on.

162

Sten Forshufvud, the twentieth-century toxicologist/detective who wrote *The Murder of Napoleon*, suspected, as did many others, that Napoleon was poisoned during his exile. The suspicion of Napoleon's fans lingered, despite an autopsy performed on the ex-emperor's corpse with the assistance of seven doctors. Four clashing autopsy reports were released. The doctors could not agree upon the cause of Napoleon's death. The British were between a rock and a hard spot. If Napoleon died from anything other than natural physical deterioration, the world would consider the former French conqueror "murdered" by his British foes. A martyr was the last thing either the British or the reinstated French monarchy wanted, for in the eyes of many Frenchmen, Napoleon was still a national military hero and statesman.

Since the autopsy found Napoleon had a gastric ulcer and *possible* cancerous tumor in his stomach, word came back from Saint Helena that Napoleon died from the Big C. Of course, none of his major symptoms—persistent gain, not loss, of weight; a yellow cast to his skin; swelling of his ankles; *and* a penis that had shrunk to an inch in length and atrophied testicles—jibed with Napoleon's being a victim of cancer. But the British doctors let the theory ride. And none of Napoleon's faithful followers to the island knew, scientifically, how to explain their ex-emperor's death. Except one, the executor to Napoleon's will, Count Montholon.

One hundred and fifty years later, Forshufvud gathered, from many areas of the world, locks of Napoleon's hair. Back then, it was the vogue to snip a lock and give it to a dear one. In fact, before Napoleon died, he ordered that the head of his corpse be shaved so locks of his hair could be sent back to special friends in France. The Swedish toxicologist gathered eight separate locks cut during different periods of Napoleon's exile. He sent these locks to a highly sophisticated lab for analysis; the results altered history. Each lock revealed a progressive increase of arsenic content as Napoleon approached his death. Read *The Murder of Napoleon* to find out how Montholon was pinned to the poisonous murder.

Unlike strychnine, arsenic, when taken in small amounts over a period of time, is not an aphrodisiac. Just the opposite, and a deadly opposite for penis and its possessor. Now, through Forshufvud's detections, we know why Montholon bit the bullet every time his wife crawled willingly into Napoleon's bed. He dragged the ex-emperor through a long, torturous death *and* two years of watching his penis shrink *and* his testicles rot before his eyes.

The moral is: Never turn your back and then have a glass with the man you christened a cuckold.

After two centuries of sexual shame and loathing, two big guns, in separate campaigns, shot through the barriers of sexual repression. The two revolutionaries, who never met, were Havelock Ellis, who unchained the penis, and Sigmund Freud, who placed it on a throne. But the enigma, which lasts to this day, is why these two astute campaigners, who resurrected and lifted the penis to exalting heights, suffered most of their sexual lives from impotency.

Biographers tell us Ellis accepted his impotent state as a "normal" maladjustment, and Freud, a "contented" husband, took a wife who cared zilch for sex. Biographers, possibly recognizing these collapsed alibis as feeble attempts to assuage the male ego, instead diagnose Freud and Ellis as geniuses too intellectually consumed to give a twitch about doing it. Supposedly, these two geniuses—unlike most other geniuses—got their uppers from counter-attacking the philosophical, religious, and scientific assaults made on human sexuality since the age of antiquity. That sounds weird, but weirder yet is the fact that these biographers believe their diagnoses reflect a normal reaction from the two founders of sexology.

164

Freud and Ellis also shared several parallel events during their lives. The two sexologists lived during the same era (Freud in Vienna and Ellis in Britain) with a mere three years' difference in their ages. And both men died in their eighties in England during the traumatic year of 1939. Both studied for the medical profession in the early 1880s and continued to practice medicine only to further their studies in human sexual behavior. Both were essayists whose creative theories on improving the sex life of the human animal met years of ridicule from their peers.

And both geniuses married, at the age of thirty and thirty-one, women who were hazardous to their sexual health and happiness.

But Ellis, while viewed by sexual historians as the less significant of the two geniuses, took a bigger gamble on the future welfare of his sex life than did the more conservative Freud. Ellis was a virgin when he married, not by choice, but because try as he might, he was unable to get it up during coitus. At the age of twenty-five, he gave it a hearty try when he fell for the feminist author Olive Schreiner. Olive was so experienced that she made no bones about making a grab for Ellis. Little did she realize that Ellis's bone was a wishbone zapped from wishing.

Six years later, Ellis took his big gamble and married his darling downer, Edith Lees, the matron of an English girls' school. Ellis married in hopes of curing his impotency. Matron Edith married hoping it would cure her sexual preference for women. Neither found their cure. But, like the loving buddies they were, both settled for a lifetime marriage of companionship.

It was then that Ellis, curious about what he was missing, began his fifty-year study of doing it. And Edith, missing what she missed, returned to her female lovers.

Inexperienced and inept, Ellis wound up making his first lengthy essay on sexuality a study in homosexuality.

Edith, the brick, naturally volunteered to be interviewed for this study.

Ellis, in his introduction to this essay (*Sexual Inversion*), says, "I do not wish any mistake to be made. I regard sex as the central problem of life. [Amen!] . . . Sex lies at the root of life, and we can never learn to reverence life until we know how to understand sex. So, at least, it seems to me."

For a man in his impotent position you gotta give it to Ellis. He could have lowered himself even further and resorted to reading dirty books. Instead, he spent decades writing his six-volume *Studies in the Psychology of Sex*, a study of sexuality so comprehensive it has yet to be matched.

And another medal, for heroic honesty, should be pinned on this persistent, though wounded, warrior. Ellis, accepting his wife's sexual preference, turned many times to the experience of "pure love." And he was always up front with his "lover." Never bemoaning or running from his impotency, Ellis opened his life to loving relationships. And the blessing of it is that his desire for a loving relationship cured him.

True, it took a while. Ellis was sixty when he got his first firm erection while doing it—but, praise be, far from his last.

It helped that Edith, after twenty-five downer years, went the way of all flesh. For, despite being an avowed lesbian, Edith was a jealous wife. Ellis always had to stop patting what he should have been patting to pat Edith's bricktopped head.

And who was it that finally taught the cofounder of sexuality what, and how, to pat to get his long-delayed erection? An intoxicating Frenchwoman, Françoise Cyon, who had turned to Ellis, now a renowned sex therapist, for consolation and advice after two failed marriages to sexually capable but insensitive men.

And what was the "secret" maneuver used by this innovative Frenchwoman to cure Ellis of his devastating maladjustment? Françoise introduced Ellis's penis to the *unique* process of mutual masturbation rhythmically timed for expansion.

Mutual masturbation was a whole new world to Ellis, especially when done by a loving, skilled technician such as his adoring Francoise.

Once inflated by the experience of coitus, Ellis found himself revolving in a whole new world. Coition eventually altered the thrust in his creative career, because in his latter years Ellis switched from writing tomes about doing it to writing brainy essays on art and literature.

Perhaps Ellis found coitus a more penetrating influence than elucidating theories on doing it. One sign pointing in that direction was his fondness in his later years for quoting his first "lover" Olive's recipe for the creation of a brainstorm. "When a man puts his penis into a woman's vagina, it is as if he put his finger into her brain, stirred it round and round. Her whole nature is affected."

If biographers of Sigmund Freud are correct, the discoverer of sexual repression knew only too well the hell of which he wrote. Freud, like Ellis, was a virgin when married at the age of thirty. But, unlike Ellis, Freud's ability to father six children during his first nine years of marriage was proof aplenty that he was more than capable of doing it. Yet, mysteriously, fifteen years after losing his virginity, Freud lost forever a most valuable treasure, his libido.

Libidos are precious things. And who would know that better than Freud, since, as the cofounder of sexology, he claimed psychiatric symptoms were the result of a misdirected or inadequate discharge of libido.

But how could a medical genius who based his analytic theories on freedom from sexual repression *and* freedom of sexual expression write a letter at the virile age of forty-one, saying "Sexual excitation is of no use to a person like me."?

What was the cause of Freud's premature impotency? Even more quizzical, why was this genius content with his soft spot below the waist when he didn't suffer from a soft spot in the head? There are many theories.

Freud claimed his loss of libido occurred because his wife (whom he loved for forty years) lost all interest in sex after bearing six children. Some analytical biographers claim Freud's impotency stemmed from a latent homosexuality. Latent only in performance, since the genius himself recognized a "leaning" toward homosexuality in his dealings with some of his male colleagues. One relationship certainly smells of it, since Freud developed a compulsive tie that lasted for several years with his eye, ear, and nose doctor, Wilhelm Fliess. Fliess also was the originator of a unique theory—that there was a direct link between the mucous membrane of the nose and genital activities.

Other clever biographers claim Freud's lack of libido is the typical trademark of a genius. These clever ones ignore such fornicating wizards as Julius Caesar, Pablo Picasso, Alexandre Dumas, Paul Gauguin, Fyodor Dostoyevski, Ernest Hemingway, Gustave Flaubert, André Gide, and Guy de Maupassant (a genius who could elevate his member on instant command).

Though few biographers mention it, Freud's addiction (for years) to cocaine was probably the downer that even this sexual genius couldn't whip.

But the biggest bone of contention is yet to come—the survival of the penis as it explodes into the twenty-first century.

12

THE PENIS EXPLODES INTO THE TWENTY-FIRST CENTURY

The twentieth century saw the rise of an explosive new penis symbol. If the penis had buttons it would burst because this expansive symbol defied the laws of gravity and opened up a universe swimming with countless new worlds. There is no denying that the aerodynamic design of the spaceship is a corker since it mimics an object so perfect—and positive—in conception that it transcends everything else on our globe.

It is almost eerie to observe a spaceship blast its way into the mystery of outer space as it echoes the male organ, with its inquisitive, exploratory head, spurred by the wonder of expansion to penetrate the limitless world of the female vagina.

Let's investigate the future of the penis on this tiny globe we call Earth, starting with the scientific and medical innovations that engender nonsexual reproduction.

If the penis should make a stand against these technologies it best be prepared to go to bat on many fronts because even now there is a lengthy list of substitutes and avoidances: artificial insemination, embryo transplants, the artificial womb, frozen germ cells, genetic engineering, in vitro fertilization, surrogate mothers, and the weirdo—asexual cloning.

If the decision is to retreat from the new facts of life, the male member could be headed the way of all flesh. Before that dire eventuality, it might be enlightening to research what's happened to breeding animals—where the bestiality of beasts can no longer be used as a moral argument against sex.

The Father of the Art of Artificial Insemination and the discoverer of nonsexual reproduction was (you might have guessed) a biologist wrapped in the robes of a Jesuit priest, the Abbé Lazzaro Spallanzani. In 1776 this Italian religious scientist challenged the biological theory that all fertilization occurs inside the female's body. (He also had the balls to tag spermatozoa "inessential parasites.") Determined to prove that life could be created outside of the womb, Abbé grabbed 165 female frogs during their sex-creative embrace with male frogs. He sliced open these hapless females, removed their eggs, and placed the ova in pond water, where they died and rotted—like mama.

Next, the inventive Abbé fashioned "little breeches of oilskin" and popped them on to male frogs about to go a courting. Still no luck.

Then this deviant biologist spread the semen trapped inside the "breeches" onto the ova of female frogs—who were probably ready to croak him when they discovered Abbé had breeched the barrier of nonsexual reproduction. And did the good Father stop at frogs? No way, for in 1780 the Abbé injected a bitch in heat with a syringe loaded with semen from a panting male dog. In sixty-two days, the bitch gave birth to three pups, each with a smarting resemblance to papa.

In humans the syringe replaced the penis in 1884 when a doctor in Philadelphia injected the unsuspecting wife of an infertile husband with semen from "the best-looking male" in the doctor's medical class. This undercover operation was not revealed until 1909 when another student from the same class, with the unreal monicker of Dr. Hard, published the facts to support his eugenic argument that this was a great technique for improving the human race.

But back to the breeding of beasts. Artificial insemination and superovulation—a process in which the female is injected with hormones to stimulate the production of ova—have been considered for years a "natural process" for improving stock, such as cattle, sheep, birds, horses, dogs, and cats. A breeder, employing these methods, claims he gets stock not only in greater quantity but of better quality.

Of quantity there is no argument—except for those who are suspicious of the ingestion of questionable hormones. Of quality there is a problem—the myth of telegony, "the influence of the sire to the offspring, and subsequent matings of the female" (*Webster*). For years animal breeders have adhered to the belief that a prize female can be ruined by a single mating with an inferior male.

Telegony was discovered/invented by Aristotle. The ancient Greek philosopher proclaimed that heredity was passed down by the male, via a sperm so potent that once a female was impregnated, *all* her offspring would carry the imprint of a previous sire.

Like all fishy stories, this one surfaced year after year. *Britannica* tells us, "An ancient English law holds a man who seduces the wet nurse of the heir to the throne guilty of polluting the 'blood' of the royal family." If so, sperm in old

England had to get a wiggle on, for it to swim upstream, exit the vagina, scoot through the womb, take a deep breath, then tackle the circuitous streams of the large and the upper intestines, and then sidestroke over to a breast. Exiting the breast, it no doubt slid down into the mouths of babes. And out of the mouths of babes, we get another fish story.

In 1868, Darwin reported with a straight face that telegony had to be legit, since he personally knew of a mare mated to a zebra and later mated to an Arabian stallion that conceived a foal with stripes on its legs.

Today breeders faithfully record their animals' credentials, especially in cases of artificial insemination.

Sperm is becoming a serious commodity, one so precious it is stored in banks. Animal sperm banks keep better accounts than human sperm banks. In animal banking procedures, all depositors must verify their past and future worth before getting an ID number. Withdrawal of sperm is debited and credited to those in charge of futures (i.e., zookeepers hoping to reduce the heredity slide due to inbreeding of animals in captivity or stockholders hoping to salvage those animals and birds on the endangered-species list).

In contrast, human sperm banking procedures are unpredictable and shockingly lax. Depositors of sperm need no verification of past or future worth (with one exception which will be computed later), no IDs, and debits and credits for withdrawals are left to dangle. For instance, in human sperm banking it is possible for a male depositor, after a withdrawal, to screw up a balance sheet. (One example: an indiscriminate sperm bank could use the sperm from one depositor to father a boy in one family and a girl in another. Later boy meets girl, they marry, then have kids who get short-changed out of their lawful genetic inheritance.) Essentially, nonsexual reproduction works in the animal world because sperm banking is carefully monitored. In humans, however, nonsexual reproduction, though not as widely used, frequently lacks documentation and, therefore, the accounting lapses.

Judging from the fact that one hundred males are conceived for every ninety-four females (this counts births, miscarriages, and abortions), more males make it being made than females. To understand why, we'll have to look at Mother Nature's recipe for making boy babies and girl babies.

Baby girls are not made of sugar and spice and everything nice. They are made of an X chromosome from the egg and an X chromosome from the sperm. These two Xs, mixed together, make a girl. And little boys are not made of snips and snails and puppy-dog tails. Their recipe calls for one X chromosome from the egg and one Y chromosome from the sperm. Mix the X and the Y together and you make a boy. (Except when making boy and girl butterflies, fishes, and birds—then the recipe is reversed.)

Selecting the sex of a child has always intrigued man—and woman. If the ingredients for making a boy were known by primitive man, who knows where we might all be now—probably still on the shelf, waiting to be mixed. Primitive man needed muscle. And primitive females were, as opposed to now, a more perishable item than the opposite sex. Female perishability was due to persistent pregnancy. For once ripe, a female was usually pregnant till the day she died—somewhere around the ripe old age of thirty. Males had their burdens to bear, but the burden of pregnancy eventually got the female.

With the coming of medical science, things took a slow switch. Now women outlive men, *but* still more males are born than females. Why, no one really knows.

But now that the recipe *and* mixing techniques are known, sex selection might be another weapon turned against the male member in the twenty-first century.

Currently, methods of sex selection are a mixed bag, and include diet, timing of ovulation and conception, straining of sperm (segregation, not strength), and vaginal foams that selectively destroy sperm. Many scientists and doctors sneer at most of these techniques despite statistics that indicate all may be partially effective. Still, all of the above echo numerous primitive folklore remedies such as eating oysters to obtain girls and salted fish to conceive boys.

In ancient India it was believed you made girl babies if there was a surfeit of menstrual blood during the menses before conception. Boys were made when there was a surfeit of male seed. But the timing had to be just right. For girl babies the forefathers of the family had to be worshiped on the second day of the vanishing moon, for boy babies the fifth day of the waning moon.

Currently some physicians claim that boy babies are made if coitus takes place during ovulation, when the environment in the cervix is alkaline and more hospitable to the less hardy male sperm. For a girl babe, coitus is timed a day or so before ovulation, when the cervix is acidic, a killer for a male-carrying sperm. The worship of the forefathers has been dropped. Replacing that ceremony is a request that your doctor's bill be paid before the moon rises on the tenth of the month.

Ancient Greeks, Romans, Jews, Slavs, and Germans claimed they could determine the sex of a babe before it was born from its position in the womb. If the fetus was curled up on the right side, it was a male; if on the left, a female.

Today science and medicine use ultrasound or amniocentesis to determine the position of the fetus and its sex. Ultrasound uses high-frequency sound waves to detect the shape and form of the body tissue. Sometimes these shapes and forms make it possible to determine the sex of the fetus. Amniocentesis is used by physicians to determine possible fetal abnormalities. In this procedure, amniotic fluid surrounding the fetus is removed and cells in the fluid examined. This examination can incidentally reveal the sex of the fetus.

Predetermination of gender before birth gives the penis an edge. In a recent Princeton survey it was discovered that both men and women suffer from feelings of penis superiority since both men and women usually prefer their first-born to be a male. If this survey proves out globally, the penis has a big edge because of a growing trend in many areas of the world for single-child families, especially in those areas which suffer from overpopulation, such as India and China. Currently the Chinese government rewards one-child families with financial benefits. Those parents who opt for more kids are taxed for each. China has yet to release statistics on the preference for a male or female child by parents in or out of this program, but it might be safe to assume the male gets the prize. In giant, overpopulated nations, girl babes strike out, for they get lower wages than men, they can't work as hard or as long, and they get pregnant.

As for the impotent male—where there's a will there's a way. Today science and medicine are on the road to abolishing impotency via penile splints, penile implants, and artificial penises.

Splints for the penis come in two models. The first is an understructure made of a flat metal core covered with rubber, and terminating, at each end, in a rubber ring. The rings come in small, medium, and large.

The limitation of three sizes makes this splint a Model-A in comparison to a more deluxe model manufactured in England by (would you believe?) Down Bros. and Mayer & Phelps Ltd. It is called the Coitus Training Apparatus (CTA). This splint is tailor-made to fit like a glove, since it is designed to accommodate any size penis. The CTA consists of two legs spread apart (not what you're thinking) and attached to the penis shaft. The head of the penis is pulled forward and a ring is attached to hold the CTA in place. A condom, not a cheap one, can be stretched over a CTA. The penis is now a lead pipe cinch.

G. Lombard Kelly, an authority on impotence, says, "Any man can use the [CTA] with satisfaction, whether he requires it full-time or not. If one is slow attaining an erection and the time for intercourse is necessarily short, the device is the answer." The device is successful in cases of premature ejaculation and the treatment of psychogenic impotence.

The artificial phallus—the penile prosthesis—is plastic and made in four sizes (average, big, bigger, and blast!). It is prescribed for those suffering from premature ejaculation or lacking a penis due to injury or disease. In itself, a plastic phallus gives sexual relief only to the partner not wearing one—a primitive device in our day of technical marvels.

The penile implant is not only primitive; it's beastly. This device ("revitalized" in Germany in 1936) made an attempt to boost the human member through a design found in nature.

Science took a peek at the privates of dogs, bears, wolves, squirrels, and whales and decided the penile bone that supported their mating activities should be extended to human males in a flap. The first operation used a section of rib cartilage to shore up an impotent male's penis. But a rib was a rib was a rib, and it didn't want to become an erection. The problems with this type of graft were that either the rib eroded out of the penis—a boggling sight—or an infection set in, putting the poor pecker in peril of amputation.

The next attempt at a penile splint stuck out like a sore thumb. In the mid-1970s a nonreactive, semirigid silicone rod was developed. The most popular of these devices was called the Small-Carrion prosthesis. This device consisted of two rods implanted in the corpora cavernosa but, one could plainly see, this device was too good to be true, for the penis was in a constant state of erection. In response, science devised a plastic rod with a hinge that was attached to the base. In action the penis was up to snuff; when the action was over, the rod packing penis was unhinged and tucked off to one side. One way or another, jockey shorts had to pull up short. Males supported by the hinged penile splint should all wear boxer shorts one size larger than their waist measurement. (They should also wear suspenders under their shirts.)

But the most flexible of all the supportive devices is the inflatable penis prosthesis devised by an American urologist in the 1970s. The device is composed of a pump, two inflatable rods, a reservoir of fluid, and tubing that connects everything. Using this system, an impotent male can produce his own erection by squeezing an inflatable bulb surgically implanted in the scrotum. The pump squeezes the fluid out of a reservoir, and the plumbing carries the fluid into the two inflatable cylinders in the cavernous bodies of the penis. The penis becomes rigid. When the time comes for a collapse, a squeeze on the bulb causes the fluid to return to its reservoir, ever ready to go onward and upward. To prove it, this device has been tested—in the laboratory—for producing erections *twice* a day for a minimum of twenty years.

Looking toward the future, science dreams of solving the mystery of total penile reconstruction and penile transplants. Once the solution is found for the problem of tissue rejection, the penis will be waiting in the wings, along with damaged hearts, livers, kidneys, brains, etc. Currently, the most assured transplant of an organ would take place between identical twins. And identical twins, of a sort, could turn out to be the Frankenstein monsters of the twenty-first century.

The problem of here today gone tomorrow might be resolved tomorrow if not today. Human cloning is considered, by some, the secret to immortality. To others, clones have a face only a mother *should* love. The "others," of whom many are scientists, claim that the cloning of humans would be a step backward for mankind. They ask us to examine: Would the world be better off if there was a plethora of Einstein brains solving the mysteries of science and mathematics? Or Freuds telling us why we act the way we do? One genius, the "others" claim, is a gift. Two, identical, redundant. Three or more identicals, a potential dictatorship.

Looking toward the future, those opposing cloning question whether an Einstein or a Freud clone will be out of sync in a future generation. A "genius in his own time" might find his days were numbered in a future environment.

Looking even further into the future, anticloners caution that the genetic pool will eventually become stagnant and could cause a stink. The *Encyclopaedia Britannica* says the "beauty" of sex is that it demands the recombination of DNA, and thus the gradual evolution of the species. With two parents this is possible—variation occurs which usually results in a "hardier" breed. Since a clone is an identical reproduction, no new mutation is possible, or at least very unlikely. Without progressive evolution, humans could open a lethal can of worms, i.e., a virus or an organism man is ill-equipped to fight off or come to terms with.

Before examining the advantages cloning has for humans, let's check out the recipe for a clone.

Clones, whether plants, animals, or microscopic organisms, are not made by—or in—sexpots. The ingredients for making a clone are so basic one might think it as easy as making apple pie. All one needs is a piece, or a single cell, of an adult being. Commercially, plants are often cloned by the process of budding, cuttings (cutting off a piece of the original plant and getting it to produce roots), and air layering (where one plant or species is grafted onto another).

Climbing the scale to higher life forms we find invertebrates cloning themselves as easy as pie. The flatworm can duplicate itself by pinching in two; each half then regenerates the missing portion. Or the worm, if cut into many pieces, regenerates a body and head for *each* piece. Since the origin of the word *clone* comes from the Greek, meaning "throng," it might be safe to assume the ancient Greeks were staring, fish-eyed, as they chopped up worms.

The recipe for a cloned mammal was not perfected until 1979 in an experiment conducted at the University of Geneva. A nucleus of a mouse egg was surgically removed, then a nucleus of a mouse cell in the blastocyte stage (after cleavage) was inserted into the recently fertilized mouse ovum. The egg was then inserted into a surrogate mother, where it grew to term.

Scientists claim this same recipe could make a human clone. All that is lacking is the technology, since it is far more difficult to transplant a nucleus out of, and into, the human egg, due to its incredibly small size.

Technology is the ball game of the twentieth century, but fear of the unknown lurks in its shadow. For example *The American Journal of Obstetrics and Gynecology* (January 15, 1979) recorded the successful replacement of three human ova with sperm cells. After the replacement, the three "tooken" eggs cleaved after thirty hours, and by the end of three days they resembled a "mulberrylike ball." In normal fertilization, this is the stage at which the ovum enters the uterus *and* it was at this stage the experiment was discontinued, despite the fact that "there was every indication that each specimen was developing normally."

And then there are those whose own member keeps a nodding. These aging or unhealthy males favor cloning as a tool for a penis transplant. Transplanting a human penis requires the elimination of immune rejection. If clones were for real, a pecker could replace a pecker from a pack of pickled peckers. If a pecker is puny, replace it. If sagging with age, pick a young one. Bruised beyond value, pick a pinker pecker from your cloned-pecker shelf. And the beauty of it is—all those peckers are *your* pecker. The sperm is your sperm, one capable of making pecker "spare parts" or "the new you." Of course, in both instances, making a clone requires an accommodating womb, but a healthy member rarely has a problem finding, or entering, "the Gate of Life."

Still other geneticists claim the future hope for making a better man, or woman, lies in sowing more seeds that are saturated with a high-ranking Intelligence Quotient.

Ninety miles south of L.A.-la land, California, lies an underground sperm bank dedicated to giving "future children the best possible start in life." The Repository for Germinal Choice claims genes are the blueprint for life and that heritability of IQ is about seventy percent. Nicknamed the "Nobel Sperm Bank" (the Repository was originally named after Herman J. Muller, a Nobel Prize winner for his discoveries on the effects of x-rays on genes), a recipient is given the choice of sperm donated by several *exceptional* donors, each of whom is "willing to increase the distribution of genes which helped to make them outstanding in their lifetime."

The Repository, founded in 1979 by a California tycoon (who said, in a telephone interview, that he was not intellectually qualified to be a donor), is on a constant treasure hunt to find "the most superlative genes to be found."

In the first five years, only nineteen donors have met the Repository's qualifications for excellence. The sperm from these juicy donors is given in several doses over a period of time, none closer than four days after intercourse. The fluid for a future brainchild is stored underground in tanks of frozen liquid nitrogen, capable of retaining the half-life of semen for ten thousand years. Since the first baby fathered by this "genius sperm bank" was born in 1982, the world will probably be in the twenty-first century before we know if a genius can pop out of a frozen can.

Far more questionable is freezing the male member, including the body that surrounds it, and expecting it to function normally after being thawed and resuscitated (the body, not the member) centuries after burial in a "Forever Flask." The process, tagged cryonics, and its philosophy—a better life after death, *if* you get properly wrapped—smacks of the ancient Egyptian funeral rituals that sought to prepare one for life in a hereafter.

For example: You have to be, like a pharaoh, loaded with dough. The cost, in the 1960s, before inflation, ran about $50,000. This does not include a bank vault (Swiss?) filled with negotiable treasures to tide one over after coming unwrapped. The corpse is wrapped from top to toe (not, God forbid, in those tacky rags used for mummies) in the cloth of the twentieth century, aluminum foil. Gleaming like a jewel, the corpse is lowered into its sophisticated sarcophagus, the Forever Flask, where it is preserved until the time is ripe to begin a new and better life. Unless the money runs out, or your tomb is robbed.

Cryonics is also used, successfully, to preserve human organs. The inventory sheet does not include the male member, but you can rest assured one is tucked away somewhere, just dying to be resuscitated.

The process for cryonics was developed out of the technology used for fueling spacecraft (low-temperature fuels such as liquid nitrogen, oxygen, and hydrogen). But, for the nonce, sex in space is a flop. The only recorded attempt was made in 1979 by the Soviet Union when they flew some spaced-out rats who refused to mate.

Still, the male member, via the spacecraft's dynamic design as a penis symbol, is on the rise. Despite gravity, the penis symbol has exploded into the universe. It has already popped up on the moon.

The fireworks have just begun.

BIBLIOGRAPHY

Anonymous. *My Secret Life*. New York: Grove Press, 1966.

Asimov, I. *Asimov's Guide to the Bible*. New York: Avenel Books, 1981.

Attenborough, D. *Life on Earth*. Boston: Little, Brown, & Co., 1979.

Barraclough, G. *The Christian World*. New York: Harry N. Abrams, 1980.

Bell, A. P., M. S. Winberg, and S. K. Hamersmith. *Sexual Preference*. Bloomington, Indiana: Indiana University Press, 1981.

Belliveau, F., and L. Richter. *Understanding Human Sexual Inadequacy*. New York: Bantam Books, 1970.

Berrill, N. J. *Sex and the Nature of Things*. New York: Dodd, Mead & Co., 1953.

Birnkrant, R. *Fascinating Facts about Love, Sex, & Marriage*. New York: Crown Publishers, 1982.

Boswell, J. *Christianity, Social Tolerance, and Homosexuality*. Chicago: University of Chicago Press, 1981.

Boyd, L. M. *Boyd's Book of Odd Facts*. New York: Signet Books, New American Library, 1979.

Brake, M., ed. *Human Sexual Relations*. New York: Pantheon Books, 1982.

Brecher, E. *The Sex Researchers*. Boston: Little, Brown & Co., 1969.

Bristow, A. *The Sex Life of Plants*. New York: Holt, Rinehart and Winston, 1978.

Brown, G. *The New Celibacy*. New York: Ballantine Books, 1980.

Brusendorf, O., and P. Henningsen. *The Complete History of Eroticism*. Secaucus, New Jersey: Castle Publishing, 1961.

Bullough, V. L. *Sexual Variance in Society and History*. Chicago: University of Chicago Press, 1976.

Bullough, V. L., and B. Bullough. *Sin, Sickness, and Sanity: A History of Sexual Attitudes*. New York: New American Library, 1977.

Calderone, M. S., and E. W. Johnson. *The Family Book about Sexuality*. New York: Harper & Row, 1981.

Casson, L. *Ancient Egypt*. New York: Time-Life Books, 1965.

Chesebro, J. W., ed. *Gayspeak: Gay Male/Lesbian Communication*. New York: Pilgrim Press, 1981.

Cole, W. G. *Sex and Love in the Bible*. New York: Associated Press, 1959.

Comfort, A., ed. *The Joy of Sex*. New York: Crown Publishers, 1972.

Comfort, A., ed. *More Joy*. New York: Crown Publishers, 1973.

Cuppy, W. *The Decline and Fall of Practically Everybody*. New York: Dell Books, 1950.

Davenport, J. *Curiosities of Erotic Physiology*. New York: Robin Hood House, 1933.

De Sade, Marquis. *The 120 Days of Sodom and Other Writings*. Compiled and translated by A. Wainhouse and R. Seaver. New York: Grove Press, 1966.

Devereaux, C. *Venus in India*. Los Angeles: Holloway House Publishing Co., 1967.

The Diagram Group. *Man's Body: An Owner's Manual*. New York: Bantam Books, 1979.

The Diagram Group. *Sex: A User's Manual*. New York: Berkley Books, 1983.

Dickinson, R. L., and L. A. Beam. *A Thousand Marriages*. Baltimore: Williams & Wilkins Co., 1931.

Douglas, N., and P. Slinger. *Sexual Secrets: The Alchemy of Ecstasy*. New York: Destiny Books, 1979.

Dunkell, S. *Lovelives*. New York: Signet Books, 1978.

Edinger, E. F. *Ego and Archetype*. Baltimore: Penguin Books, 1973.

Edwards, P., ed. *The Encyclopedia of Philosophy*. Vols. 1–8. New York: Macmillan Publishing Co., 1972.

Ellis, A., and A. Abarbanel, ed. *The Encyclopedia of Sexual Behavior*. New York: Jason Aronson, 1973.

Ellis, A. *Sex Without Guilt*. New York: Lyle Stuart, 1958.

Ellis, H. *Psychology of Sex*. 2nd ed. New York: Harcourt, Brace & Jovanovich, 1966.

Ellis, H. *Studies in the Psychology of Sex*. Vols. 1 and 2. New York: Random House, 1942.

Ellison, A. *Sex between Humans and Animals*. Vol. 2. San Diego: Academy Press, 1970.

Finch, B. E., and H. Green. *Contraception through the Ages*. London: Peter Owen, 1963.

Fischer, L. *The Life of Mahatma Gandhi*. New York, Collier, 1966.

Fisher, H. *The Sex Contract*. New York: William Morrow & Co., 1982.

Fisher, P. *The Gay Mystique*. New York: Stein and Day, 1972.

Flaceliere, R., trans. *Love in Ancient Greece*. Westport: Greenwood Press, 1973.

Flaubert, G. *The Letters of Gustave Flaubert, 1830–1857*. F. Steegmuller, trans. Cambridge: The Belknap Press of Harvard University Press, 1980.

Foucault, M. *The History of Sexuality*. Vol. 1. New York: Vintage House, 1980.

Francoen, R. T. *Utopian Motherhood: New Trends in Human Reproduction*. Garden City: Doubleday & Co., 1970.

Frazer, Sir J. G. *The Golden Bough*. Vol. 1, abridged. New York: Macmillan Publishing Co., 1963.

Freedman, H. *Sex Link*. New York: M. Evans & Co., 1977.

Freud, S. *Three Essays on the Theory of Sexuality*. New York: Basic Books, 1962.

Fryer, P. *The Birth Controllers*. New York: Stein and Day, 1965.

Gadd, L., and Editors of the World Almanac. *The World Almanac— Book of the Strange*. New York: Signet Books, 1981.

Gandhi, M. K. *An Autobiography*, M. Desai, trans. Boston: Beacon Press, 1957.

Gerber, A. B., comp. *The Book of Sex Lists*. Secaucus, New Jersey: Lyle Stuart, 1981.

Gibbon, E. *The Decline and Fall of the Roman Empire*. New York: Wise & Co., 1943.

Goldberg, I. *The Sacred Fire*. New York: Alfred A. Knopf, 1930.

Gosselin, C. and G. Wilson. *Sexual Variations*. New York: Simon and Schuster, 1980.

Grant, M. *From Alexander to Cleopatra*. New York: Charles Scribner's Sons, 1982.

Grant, M. *The Twelve Caesars*. New York: Charles Scribner's Sons, 1975.

Grayzel, S. *A History of the Jews*. New York: Mentor Books, 1968.

Green, S. *The Curious History of Contraception*. New York: St. Martin's Press, 1971.

Hamilton, R. *The Herpes Book*. Los Angeles: J. B. Tarcher, 1980.

Heinrich, M. R., and K. A. Souza, ed. *Final Reports of U.S. Rat Experiments Flown on the Soviet Satellite Cosmos 1129*. NASA

Technical Memorandum 81289, Ames Research Center, Moffet Field, California, August 1981.

Himes, N. E. *Medical History of Contraception.* New York: Gamut Press, 1963.

The Hindu Art of Love (Ananga Ranga). London: Castle Books, 1969.

Hite, S. *The Hite Report on Male Sexuality.* New York: Alfred A. Knopf, 1981.

Hopper, R. J. *The Early Greeks.* New York: Barnes & Noble, 1976.

Hunt, M. M. *The Natural History of Love.* New York: Alfred A. Knopf, 1959.

Hunt, N. *Mirror Image.* New York: Holt, Rinehart and Winston, 1978.

Infield, G. B. *Secret Life: The Mysteries of the Eagle's Nest.* New York: Stein and Day, 1979.

Jones, E. *The Life and Work of Sigmund Freud.* New York: Basic Books, 1961.

Kahn, S. S. *The Kahn Report on Sexual Preferences.* New York: St. Martin's Press, 1981.

The Kama Sutra of Vatsyayana. Sir R. Burton, trans. New York: Berkley Books, 1984.

Karlen, A. *Sexuality and Homosexuality.* New York: W. W. Norton & Co., 1971.

Kavaler, L. *A Matter of Degree.* New York: Harper & Row, 1981.

Kiefer, O. *Sexual Life in Ancient Rome.* New York: Barnes & Noble, 1962.

Kinsey, A. C., W. Pomeroy, C. E. Martin, and P. H. Gebhard. *Sexual Behavior of the Human Female.* Philadelphia: W. B. Saunders, 1953.

Kinsey, A. C., W. Pomeroy, C. E. Martin, and P. H. Gebhard. *Sexual Behavior of the Human Female.* Philadelphia: W. B. Saunders, 1953.

Knauth, P., ed. *The Illustrated Encyclopedia of the Animal World.* New York: The Danbury Press, 1971.

Krafft-Ebing, R. V. *Psychopathia Sexualis.* F. B. Rebman, trans. New York: Physicians and Surgeons Book Co., 1934.

Kramer, S. N. *Cradle of Civilization.* New York: Time-Life Books, 1967.

Krich, A., ed. *The Sexual Revolution.* New York: Dell Books, 1963.

Kruck, W. E. *Looking for Dr. Condom.* University, Alabama: University of Alabama Press, 1981.

Legman, G. *Ora-Genitalism.* New York: Causeway Books, 1969.

Lehrman, N. *Masters & Johnson Explained.* New York: Playboy Paperbacks, 1970.

Lindsay, R. *How to Look as Young as You Feel.* Los Angeles: Pinnacle Books, 1980.

Ludwig, E. *Napoleon.* New York: Liveright, 1954.

"M." *The Sensuous Man.* New York: Dell Books, 1971.

McKale, D. M. *Hitler: The Survival Myth.* New York: Stein and Day, 1981.

Malinowski, B. *Sex, Culture, and Myth.* London: Hart-Davis, 1963.

Malinowski, B. *The Sexual Life of Savages.* New York: Harcourt, Brace & World, 1929.

Marcus, S. *The Other Victorians.* New York: Meridian Books, 1974.

Marvels and Mysteries of Our Animal World. Pleasantville, New York: The Reader's Digest Association, 1964.

Masson, J. M. *The Assault on Truth: Freud's Suppression of the Seduction Theory.* New York: Farrar, Straus and Giroux, 1984.

Masters, W. H., and V. E. Johnson. *Human Sexual Response.* Boston: Little, Brown & Co., 1966.

Masters, W. H., and V. E. Johnson. *The Pleasure Bond.* New York: Bantam Books, 1980.

Mead, M. *Male and Female.* New York: Morrow Quill Paperbacks, 1977.

Meyer, J. J. *Sexual Life in Ancient India.* New York: Barnes & Noble, 1953.

Moore, H., and J. W. Barrett, ed. *Who Killed Hitler?* New York: The Booktab Press, 1947.

Moore, J. C. *Love in Twelfth Century France.* Philadelphia: University of Pennsylvania Press, 1972.

Morris, D. *Animal Days.* New York: Perigord Press, 1979.

Morris, D. *Manwatching.* New York: Harry N. Abrams, 1977.

Morris, D. *The Naked Ape.* New York: McGraw-Hill, 1967.

Morris, I. *The Pillow Book of Sei Shonagon.* New York: Penguin Books, 1971.

The New Larousse Encyclopedia of Animal Life. New York: Bonanza Books, 1980.

Newman, F. X., ed. *The Meaning of Courtly Love.* Albany, New York: State University of New York Press, 1968.

Parrinder, G., ed. *World Religions.* New York: Facts on File, 1983.

Partridge, E. *Origins.* New York: Macmillan Publishing Co., 1966.

Penny, A. *How to Make Love to a Man*. New York: Dell Publishing, 1982.

The Perfumed Garden of the Shaykh Nefzawi. Sir R. Burton, trans. New York: Gramercy Publishing, 1963.

Pfeiffer, J. E. *The Creative Explosion*. New York: Harper & Row, 1982.

Pietropinto, A., and J. Simenauer. *Beyond the Male Myth*. New York: Signet Books, 1977.

Raley, P. E. *Making Love*. New York: Dial Press, 1976.

Rawson, H. *A Dictionary of Euphemisms and Other Doubletalk*. New York: Crown Publishers, 1981.

Reuben, D. *Everything You Always Wanted to Know about Sex*. New York: Bantam Books, 1980.

Ropp, R. S. *Sex Energy*. New York: Delta Books, 1969.

Sanger, W. *The History of Prostitution*. New York: Eugenics Publishing Co., 1937.

Scott, G. R. *Curious Customs of Sex & Marriage*. London: Torchstream Books, 1953.

Schulberg, L. *Historic India*. New York: Time-Life Books, 1968.

Seligmann, K. *Magic, Supernaturalism and Religion*. New York: Pantheon Books, 1971.

Shipley, J. T. *Dictionary of Word Origins*. New York: The Philosophical Library, 1945.

Silber, S. J. *The Male*. New York: Charles Scribner's Sons, 1981.

Spears, R. A. *Slang and Euphemism*. Middle Village, New York: Jonathan David Publishers, 1981.

Stebbins, G. *Darwin to DNA, Molecules to Humanity*. New York: W. H. Freeman and Co., 1982.

Stern, M. *Sex in the USSR*. M. Howson, C. Ryan, trans. and ed. New York: Times Books, 1980.

Tannahill, R. *Sex in History*. New York: Stein and Day, 1980.

Taylor, G. R. *Sex in History*. New York: Harper Torchbooks, 1970.

Terres, J. K. *The Audubon Society Encyclopedia of North American Birds*. New York: Alfred A. Knopf, 1980.

Thompson, P. *The Edwardians*. New York: Paladin Books, 1975.

Toland, J. *Adolf Hitler*. New York: Ballantine Books, 1977.

Toynbee, A. J. *A Study of History*. New York: Oxford University Press, 1947.

Trevor-Roper, H. R. *The Last Days of Hitler*. New York: Macmillan Publishing Co., 1947.

Wallace, I., A. Wallace, D. Wallechinsky, and S. Wallace. *The Intimate Sex Lives of Famous People*. New York: Delacorte Press, 1981.

Wallace, R. A. *How They Do It*. New York: Quill Paperbacks, 1980.

Walters, R. G., ed. *Primers for Prudery*. Englewood Cliffs, New Jersey: Prentice-Hall, 1974.

Walton, A. H. *Aphrodisiacs: From Legend to Prescription*. Westport, Connecticut: Associated Booksellers, 1958.

Wedeck, H. E. *Dictionary of Aphrodisiacs*. New York: Philosophical Library, 1961.

Weider, B., and D. Hapgood. *The Murder of Napoleon*. New York: Berkley Books, 1983.

Weinberg, M. S., and C. J. Williams. *Male Homosexuals*. New York: Oxford University Press, 1974.

Wendt, H. *The Sex Life of Animals*. New York: Simon and Schuster, 1965.

Wilson, C., ed. *Dark Dimensions*. New York: Everest House, 1977.

Young, W. *Eros Denied: Sex in Western Society*. New York: Grove Press, 1964.

INDEX

abstinence, 74–91
Acton, William, 25, 50
adrenal glands, 107
Agrippina, 82
AIDS (Acquired Immune
    Deficiency Syndrome),
    129–130
Ai Tai, Emperor of China, 143
Aleksey Nikolaevich,
    Tsarevich of Russia, 156,
    157
Alexander VI, Pope, 89–90 ~
Ambrose, Saint, 83
*American Journal of Obstetrics
    and Gynecology*, 179
*American Journal of Public
    Health*, 112
American Social Health
    Association, 128
amniocentesis, 174–175
amphetamines, 73
Ananga Ranga, 2
androgen, 105
animals, 13–15, 30–31, 33–35,
    65–67, 107–108, 110, 132,
    140
Antony, Marc, 81
anus, 16, 22, 101, 111, 130
Aphrodisia, 56
aphrodisiacs, 54–73
Aphrodite, 62–63
Archibald, George, 66–67

armadillos, 14
Ars Amatoria (Ovid), 38
artificial insemination,
    170–173
Asimov, Isaac, 56
Asimov's Guide to the Bible
    (Asimov), 56
Augustine, Saint, 18–19, 83,
    84–86
autofellatio, 30
autosexuals, 16

barbiturates, 72
Barham, Patte, 159
Basil, Saint, 83–84
bats, 13–14
Baudelaire, Charles-Pierre,
    118
bears, 30
bedbugs, 34
bees, 59–60
Beethoven, Ludwig van, 117
Behan, Brendan, 151, 155
Bell, Alan P., 131
Bible, 49–50, 56, 60–61, 144
Binet, Alfred, 64
Borgia, Cesare, 90, 118
Borgia, Lucrezia, 90
Borgia, Rodrigo, 89–90
Bormann, Martin, 153, 154
Borstal Boy (Behan), 151, 155
Boswell, John, 142, 143

Braun, Eva, 152, 153, 154
Brecher, Edward M., 125
Bristow, Alec, 58
Bronze Age, phallic symbolism
    in, 17
Buddhism, 76
bulls, 14
Burton, Sir Richard, 4–5
Byrnes, James F., 153–154

Caelius Aurelianus, 142–143
Caesar, Gaius Julius, 142, 168
Calvin, John, 90
cantharis, 71–72
Capone, Al, 118
Cary, Henry N., 45
castration, 92–108
Cellini, Benvenuto, 117
Centers for Disease Control,
    130
Charles II, King of England,
    119
Charles VII, King of France,
    147
Charles VIII, King of France,
    112–113, 117
Cheng Ho, 96–97
Chesebro, James W., 132
chimpanzees, 34–35
China, 37, 39–41, 58, 69–70
Christianity, 19, 20, 22–23, 28,
    29, 37, 50, 80–87, 143
*Christianity Social Tolerance
    and Homosexuality*
    (Boswell), 142, 143
Churchill, Randolph, Lord,
    117
City of Hope, The (Augustine),
    85–86
Cleopatra VII, Queen of Egypt,
    81
cloning, 177–179
cocaine, 70–71, 72
coitus reservatus, 48–49

Columbus, Christopher,
    113–114, 117
Columbus, Ferdinand, 113
*Compact Edition of the Oxford
    English Dictionary, The*, 6
condoms, 118–122, 125, 127,
    176
Cook, James, 117
coprolalia, 68
copulation, 13–15, 38–46, 49,
    51
Cowper's glands, 51
cryonics, 181
cunnilingus, 41
Cuppy, Will, 82
Custer, George, 118

Dante Alighieri, 87
Darius I, King of Persia, 94
Dark Dimensions (Wilson),
    157–158
Darwin, Charles, 172
*Decline and Fall of Practically
    Everybody, The* (Cuppy), 82
*Decline and Fall of the Roman
    Empire, The* (Gibbon), 142
de Isla, Ruy Diaz, 114
De Morbo Gallico (Fallopius),
    118
de Sade, Marquis, 64, 71, 117
Devereaux, Charles, 5–6
Dictionary of Aphrodisiacs, The
    (Wedeck), 55, 72
dogs, 30, 31
Dönitz, Karl, 153
Donizetti, Gaetano, 117
Dostoyevski, Fyodor, 168
Douglas, Alfred, Lord, 149
Douglas, Nik, 3
dragonflies, 13
Drysdale, Charles, 25
Dumas, Alexandre, 118, 168
Durant, Will, 79, 87

Egypt, ancient, 17, 21–22, 120, 132
Eisenhower, Dwight D., 153
ejaculation, 5, 14, 25, 26, 49, 53
Eleanor of Aquitaine, 87–88
elephants, 30
Ellis, Havelock, 26, 36–37, 61–62, 141, 149, 164–167
Encyclopaedia Britannica, 74–75, 97, 155, 178
Encyclopedia of Sexual Behavior (Ellis and Abarbanel, eds.), 54, 101, 110
Erasmus, Desiderius, 118
erections, 1–3, 5, 13–15, 18, 51, 53, 54, 61–62, 73, 175–177
erogenous zones, 33
Erroneous Turns of the Sex Drive, The (Fleck), 24
estrogen, 105
excitement phase, 51

Fallopius, Gabriel, 118
fellatio, 30, 41, 62
fetishism, 64–67
flagellation, 62–64
Flaubert, Gustave, 92–93, 98, 168
fleas, 15
Fleck, Johann, 24
Fliess, Wilhelm, 168
Forshufvud, Sten, 162–164
Fracastoro, Girolamo, 115–116
Francis Ferdinand, Archduke of Austria, 157
Frauendienst (Lichtenstein), 88–89
Freud, Sigmund, 19, 91, 164, 167–168
Fülöp-Miller, René, 156

Galen, 109–110
Gandhi, Harilal, 77
Gandhi, Mohandas K., 77
Gauguin, Paul, 117, 168
Gautama Buddha, 76
genital herpes, 125–129
Gibbon, Edward, 142
Gide, André, 168
Gilles de Rais, 147–148
ginseng, 58
goats, 30
Goddess of the Shell, 40–41
Goebbels, Joseph, 153, 154
Goebbels, Magda, 153, 154
Goethe, Johann Wolfgang von, 117–118
gonorrhea, 109–112, 122–123, 124–125, 126
Goodyear, Charles, 121
gorillas, 14, 30, 34
Goya, Francisco José de, 117
graffiti, sexual, 35
Graham, Sylvester, 26
Greece, ancient, 18, 21, 56, 60, 62–63, 77–79, 140–142, 143

Hamburger, Christian, 104
Hamilton, Richard, 127–128
Hannibal, 94
Haydn, Franz Joseph, 98
Hemingway, Ernest, 168
hermaphrodites, 101
heroin, 69–70, 72
herpes, genital, 125–129
Herpes Book, The (Hamilton), 127–128
Herpes Resource Center, 126
Hickok, James Butler "Wild Bill," 118
Hijras, 101
Hinduism, 76, 77, 101
Hippocrates, 107
Hirshfield, Magnus, 149

History of Prostitution, A
    (Sanger), 114–115
Hite, Shere, 29
Hite Report on Male Sexuality,
    The (Hite), 29
Hitler, Adolf, 151–155
Hitler, Eva Braun, 152, 153,
    154
homosexuality, 34, 79, 99, 111,
    131–150, 165–166
homunculi, 52
horses, 107–108
How They Do It (Wallace), 14
humpback whales, 14

impotency, 54, 55, 70–71, 73,
    175–177
imprinting, 65–67
India, 76–77, 101, 174
Indians, American, 113, 117
Islam, 21, 92–93, 98–99

Jacobi, Abraham, 27
Jainism, 76–77
Jalade-Lafond, G., 24
Japan, condoms in, 121
Jerome, Saint, 83
Jesus, 96
Joan of Arc, 147, 148
John, Saint, 95–96
Johnson, Virginia E., 49,
    51–52
Jorgensen, George (Christine),
    103–104
Josephine, Empress of France,
    160, 161
Journal of the American
    Medical Association, 123
Joyce, James, 118
Judaism, 17–18, 21, 29, 49–50,
    79–80, 90, 143, 144
Julius II, Pope, 118

Kama Sutra (Vatsyayana), 2–3,
    38–39, 41

kangaroos, 13
Kaposi's sarcoma, 129
Karo, Joseph, 80
Keats, John, 117
Kellogg, John Harvey, 26–27
Kelly, G. Lombard, 176
Kinsey, Alfred C., 28, 29–31,
    34, 35, 45, 108
Kinsey Institute for Research,
    45
kissing, 35–38
Knights Templar, 145–146
Krafft-Ebing, Richard Freiherr
    von, 26, 63, 149
Krishna, 17, 101

Ladies Home Journal, 46
Lees, Edith, 165–166
Legman, G., 41
Liber, 18, 19
Liberalis, Antoninus, 120
Lichtenstein, Ulrich von,
    88–89
Life of Greece, The (Durant), 79
Linga Purana, 5
lizards, 15
lobsters, 15
LSD, 72
Luther, Martin, 89

Magellan, Ferdinand, 117
Male, The (Silber), 5
mandrake, 56–57, 61
marijuana, 54, 72
masochism, 62–64
Masters, William H., 49, 51–52
masturbation, 20–31, 75, 167
Maupassant, Guy de, 118, 168
Medical Aspects of Human
    Sexuality, 51
Melicow, M. M., 98
Minos, 120
Molay, Jacques de, 146
Montesquieu, 100

Montholon, Albine de, 160–162
Montholon, Charles-Tristan de, 160–162, 163–164
Morris, Desmond, 66
mosquitoes, 13
Muller, Herman J., 180
multiple penises, 15, 17
Murder of Napoleon, The (Forshufvud), 162–164
Musmanno, Michael, 154
Mussolini, Benito, 117
Myers, Lonny, 3, 122–125

Napoleon I, Emperor of France, 64, 98, 117, 148, 160–164
Napoleonic Code, 148, 161
narcissism, 16
National Association of Broadcasters, 121–122
Natural History of Love, The (Hunt), 83, 89
Nazirites, 80
Neolithic era, phallic symbolism in, 16
Nero, Emperor of Rome, 57, 82, 94
New Celibacy, The (Brown), 91
New Standard Dictionary, 75
New York Times Index, 155
Nicholas II, Tsar of Russia, 156, 157, 158
Nietzsche, Friedrich Wilhelm, 118

octopi, 15, 34
Onan, 49
One Thousand and One Sexual Embraces, 39
On Onanism (Tissot), 23
opium, 69–70
Ora-Genitalism (Legman), 41
oral sex, 30, 41, 62
orchids, 57, 58–60

orgasmic phase, 51–52
orgasms, 51–53
Origins (Partridge), 33
Orphism, 78
Osiris, 17
Ovid, 38
Oxford English Dictionary, The Compact Edition of, 6

Pacion, Stanley J., 77
Paracelsus, 116–117
Partridge, Eric, 33
Paul, Saint, 80–82, 97
PCP *(Pneumocystis carinii pneumonia)*, 129
penguins, 34
penile implants, 54, 73, 175–177
Perfumed Garden, The, 4–5, 61
Perkins, Miss, 27
Persian Letters (Montesquieu), 100
Peter I, Tsar of Russia, 117
Petronius, 57
Phaedo (Plato), 78
Phaedrus (Plato), 79
phallic symbolism, 16–19
Philip II, King of Spain, 117
Philip IV, King of France, 146
Philip V, King of Spain, 98
Philo Judaeus, 144–145
Picasso, Pablo, 168
pigs, 14
plateau phase, 51
Plato, 78–79
Plemme, Thomas E., 72
Pliny, 57
poppy, 69–70
porcupines, 14–15, 30, 34, 35
pornography, 5–6, 16, 35, 38, 55, 62
postcoital disinfection, 123, 125
Prayer Cushion of the Flesh, The, 3

premature ejaculation, 49
Prepared Table, The (Karo), 80
priapism, 18
Priapus, 18
prostitutes, 63, 64, 105, 112, 125
psychedelic drugs, 72
Psychopathia Sexualis (Krafft-Ebing), 26
Ptolemy Philadelphus, King of Egypt, 17
Public Health Service, U.S., 111

Queensberry, John Sholto Douglas, Marquess of, 148–149

race, penis size and, 3
Rasputin, Grigori, 155–160
Rasputin, Maria, 159
Repository for Germinal Choice, 180
reptiles, 15
rhinoceroses, 14
Richard I, King of England, 87
Rome, ancient, 18–19, 36–37, 57–58, 60, 94–95

Sacher-Masoch, Ritter Leopold von, 63
Sade, Marquis de, 64, 71, 117
sadism, 64
Sanger, William 114–115
Satyricon, The (Petronius), 57
satyrion, 57
satyrs, 57
Schopenhauer, Arthur, 118
Schreiner, Olive, 165, 167
Schumann, Robert, 117
Scythians, 107–108
seahorses, 15
self-fellatio, 30
semen, 2, 3, 14, 21, 47–53, 60

Sensuous Man, The (M), 37–38
Sex in History (Tannahill), 95
Sex Life of Plants, The (Bristow), 58
Sex Researchers, The (Brecher), 125
sex selection and determination, 173–175
Sexual Behavior of the Human Female (Kinsey), 34
Sexual Inversion (Ellis), 166
Sexual Secrets (Douglas), 3
Sexual Variance (Acton), 50, 83–84, 101
Shaker movement, 90–91
Silber, Sherman J., 5
size, penile, 1–3, 13–15
Slang and Euphemism (Spears), 21
Smith, David E., 70
snakes, 15
Socrates, 78
Song of Solomon, 56, 80
Soranus, 142–143
Spallanzani, Abbé Lazzaro, 170–171
Spanish fly, 71–72
Sparling, P. Frederick, 122
Spears, Richard A., 21
spermatozoa, 52–53, 170–171
spermatorrhea, 25, 26
sperm banks, 172–173, 180
spiders, 15
"squeeze play" technique, 49
Stalin, Joseph, 153–154
Star of David, symbolism of, 17–18
Stendhal, 118
Stern, Mikhail, 16
Stone Age, phallic symbolism in, 16
Studies in the Psychology of Sex (Ellis), 36–37, 166
Swift, Jonathan, 36

Symposium (Plato), 79
syphilis, 112–118, 122,
123–125, 126

Tacitus, 82
tagged cryonics, 181
Talmud, 21, 80
Tannahill, Reay, 95
telegony, 171–172
telephone erotica, 68
testicles, 15, 17, 60, 92–108,
110, 151, 152, 163, 164
testosterone, 105, 107
ticks, genitalia of, 15
Tissot, S. A., 23
toads, 15
Toulouse-Lautrec, Henri de,
117
transplants, penis, 179–180
transsexuality, 67, 102,
103–106
transvestism, 67–68, 105
Trevor-Roper, Hugh, 154
Truman, Harry S, 153–154
tuataras, 15
turtles, 15

Ulrichs, Karl Heinrichs, 149
ultrasound, 174
Uranus, 149

urethra, 5
urination, 21, 105, 110
Urology, 98

vaginas, 21, 48, 60, 102,
103–104, 105–106
vajroli, 49
Varro, Marcus Terentius,
18–19
Vatican Library, 28
Vatsyayana, 38–39
Vedism, 76
venereal diseases, 109–130
Venus in India (Devereaux),
5–6
Verlaine, Paul, 118
voyeurism, 62

Wallace, Robert A., 14
Wedeck, Harry E., 55
whales, humpback, 14
Wilde, Oscar, 118, 131,
148–149
Wilson, Colin, 157–158
Wolf, Hugo, 117

yin essence, 48

Zhukov, Georgi K., 153